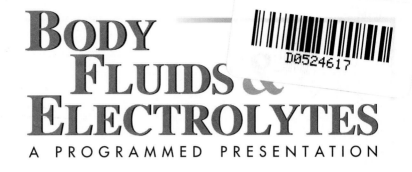

BODY
FLUIDS &
ELECTROLYTES

A PROGRAMMED PRESENTATION

BODY FLUIDS & ELECTROLYTES

A PROGRAMMED PRESENTATION

Eighth Edition

with 31 illustrations and 14 tables

ELIZABETH SPEAKMAN, Ed.D., R.N.
Associate Professor of Nursing
Community College of Philadelphia
Philadelphia, Pennsylvania

NORMA JEAN WELDY, B.S., M.S., R.N.
Professor Emerita
Goshen College
Goshen, Indiana

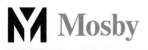 Mosby

St. Louis   London   Philadelphia   Sydney   Toronto

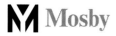

Vice President and Publishing Director, Nursing: *Sally Schrefer*
Senior Editor: *Michael Ledbetter*
Associate Developmental Editor: *Amanda Sunderman Politte*
Project Manager: *John Rogers*
Senior Production Editor: *Helen Hudlin*
Designer: *Kathi Gosche*

NOTICE
Pharmacology is an ever-changing field. Standard safety precautions must be followed, but as new research and clinical experience broaden our knowledge, changes in treatment and drug therapy may become necessary or appropriate. Readers are advised to check the most current product information provided by the manufacturer of each drug to be administered to verify the recommended dose, the method and duration of administration, and contraindications. It is the responsibility of the licensed prescriber, relying on experience and knowledge of the patient, to determine dosages and the best treatment for each individual patient. Neither the publisher nor the editor assumes any liability for any injury and/or damage to persons or property arising from this publication.

Mosby, Inc.
11830 Westline Industrial Drive
St. Louis, Missouri 63146

Printed in the United States of America

ISBN 0-323-01274-4

01 02 03 04 05 CL/RDC 9 8 7 6 5 4 3 2 1

To my children,

Alexandra and Caroline,

my husband,

Bob,

and my parents,

Robert and Betty St. John,

thank you for all the opportunities

to venture into new endeavors.

You are my inspiration.

To my sister,

Jane,

and brother,

Chris,

and to my

colleagues and students at the Community College of Philadelphia,

thank you for your

unconditional support and encouragement.

REVIEWERS

KATHLEEN G. STILLING, R.N., C., M.S.
Assistant Professor, Nursing
Community College of Baltimore
County Essex Campus
Baltimore, Maryland

CHERYL L. BRADY, R.N., M.S.N.
Adjunct Faculty
Kent State University
East Liverpool, Ohio

PREFACE

Fluid, electrolyte, and acid-base balance within the body is essential for maintaining health and function in all body systems. This text is designed to assist experienced and inexperienced nurses in understanding the complexity of fluid, electrolyte, and acid-base balance and the many clinical conditions related to an imbalance. Nurses and nursing students who have mastered a thorough knowledge of body fluids and electrolytes will be able to care for their patients by using greater critical thinking skills. Understanding that fluid, electrolyte, and acid-base imbalances may affect any individual regardless of age, sex, ethnicity, or race is essential. This book is a programmed unit that helps nurses realize that over a period of time an individual's inability to adapt adequately to these changes leads to altered health states and potential chronic health problems.

This text provides information in sequence, building from simple to complex. Each step builds on previous learning. **Key Terms** are listed at the beginning of each part to make the reader aware of terminology that is pertinent to the content in that part. **Concept Checks** are followed by **Information Checks** throughout the book. These sections are designed to help both the experienced and inexperienced nurse decide when to move on to the next section. At the end of each part, a list of **Key Points** is given, followed by a series of **Critical Thinking Questions.** New to this edition are **Remember Boxes** to emphasize need-to-know information.

Programmed material presents organized information that allows each individual to learn at his/her own pace. Classroom discussions are useful for nursing students who have completed the program. The use of case study analysis can assist students in synthesizing the various types of fluid, electrolyte, and acid-base imbalances, the signs and symptoms that can be observed, and the nursing care that is indicated. The percentages and laboratory values relate to infants, children, young and middle-aged adults, and elderly persons.

The ultimate objectives of this text are to enable the reader to:

1. Describe the basic physiological mechanisms responsible for maintaining body fluid, electrolyte, and acid-base balances.
2. Describe the distribution of body fluids and electrolytes in infants, children, adults, and elderly persons.
3. Identify major causes of body fluid, electrolyte, and acid-base imbalances and the signs and symptoms that indicate such imbalances.
4. List important assessments for a person who has, or is at high risk for, body fluid, electrolyte, or acid-base imbalance.
5. Describe nursing management for a person who has, or is at high risk for, body fluid, electrolyte, or acid-base imbalance.
6. Compare nursing assessment and management for a person with acidosis or alkalosis.
7. Examine the appropriate delegation activities.

HOW TO USE THIS PROGRAM UNIT

This is a program designed to help you understand the need for balance in body fluids, electrolytes, and acid-base. It will help define key terms necessary for understanding the complexity of body fluid, electrolyte, and acid-base balance and the mechanism by which fluids and electrolytes are moved and regulated. The reader should gain information on how body fluids and electrolytes are lost and then replaced both in health and in disease. Through this program unit, you should learn to recognize the signs and symptoms that indicate an imbalance of body fluids or electrolytes.

The program will help you recognize laboratory tests that indicate imbalance and some of the common methods of treating the imbalance. Subsequently, you should learn what is important nursing care to patients who have, or may have, an imbalance in body fluids or electrolytes. You will also understand the severity and long-term effects on the health of an individual that has been compromised by an imbalance and how it will influence that individual's ability to return to a state of optimal functioning. It is important that nurses realize that prolonged or severe complications may lead to irreversible health problems that will have an impact, not only on an individual, but on his/her family as well.

Each statement or paragraph is called a frame. At the end of each frame, there is a question with a place to respond. The answers are given in the left-hand column. As you work through the program, read carefully, and completely formulate your answers to the questions before you look at the answer given. Use the template provided to cover the answer column.

There are four types of statements to be completed:

1. Sometimes there is a blank included where you will fill in the word or phrase to correctly complete the statement. Write your answer in the blank and then compare it with the correct response in the answer column.
2. Sometimes you will need to make a choice from two or three answers. Circle the correct choice and compare your response with the answer column.
3. Some statements ask you to respond to questions or situations in your own words. Check your written answer with the suggestions made in the answer column. Your answer does not have to be identical, but it must contain the same idea.
4. Some statements ask you to select the right answers from a list of several possible answers. Make a check next to the correct answers and compare your response with the answer column.

Elizabeth Speakman
Norma Jean Weldy

CONTENTS

FLUID AND ELECTROLYTE BALANCE

INTRODUCTION

Maintaining fluid and electrolyte balance is essential for all body systems to function. People cannot live without body fluid; it is the largest single constituent of the body. In the average young to middle-aged adult, total body fluid amounts to about 55% to 60% of body weight, while, in the newborn infant, total fluid is 75% to 80% of body weight. Because the highest percentage of body weight in an infant is fluid, maintaining fluid balance is extremely important. By the age of 2 years, the percentage of body weight that is fluid is approximately the same as that of a young to middle-aged adult. In the elderly, changes in body tissues cause the total body fluid to drop to 45% to 50% of body weight. Because the elderly have a much lower percentage of body weight that is fluid, they are also highly likely to develop fluid imbalance. Therefore one of the important functions of the nurse is to assess the patient's fluid balance or imbalance.

When an individual loses fluids, by vomiting for example, some of the normal fluid content of the body is lost. If the vomiting continues and the person does not drink fluids, the loss may become serious. The individual will experience dry mucous membranes, an increase in body temperature, and may become lethargic. If the fluid loss goes untreated, over time the body's compensatory mechanisms will no longer maintain an adequate fluid balance, and the individual's health may become compromised. Depending on the severity, fluid loss can lead to irreversible health problems or death. A loss of 20% of the body's fluid content is fatal. For example, a person with third-degree burns over a major portion of the body will lose fluid through seepage from the burned areas. If the fluid is not replaced, death will occur. Replacing body fluid and managing fluid balance will decrease the risk of the harmful effects of fluid loss.

KEY TERMS

active transport
adenosine triphosphate
aldosterone
angiotensin I
angiotensin II
anion
anion gap
anode
antidiuretic hormone
cathode
cation
colloid osmotic pressure
diffusion
edema
electrolytes
electroneutrality
extracellular
filtration
homeostasis
hydrostatic pressure
hypertonic
hypotonic
insensible fluid loss
interstitial
intracellular
intravascular
isotonic
oncotic pressure
osmolality
osmolarity
osmosis
osmotic pressure
pressure gradient
renin
sensible fluid loss
solute(s)
solvent
specific gravity

1. Body fluids have two main functions. One of the functions of body fluids is to provide transportation of nutrients to cells and to carry waste products from cells.

   transportation of   One function of body fluids is to provide _____
       nutrients   _____ to cells and _____ away
   carry waste products   from cells.

2. A second major function of body fluids is to provide a medium in which electrolyte chemical reactions can occur.

   electrolyte chemical   Body fluids transport nutrients to and waste products
       reactions   from the cells, and they are also necessary so that
                          _____ can occur.

BODY FLUID COMPARTMENTS

3. Body fluids are distributed into two compartments. The word compartment is used to describe where fluid is found in the body. Most of the body fluids are inside the cells, and this is called the **intracellular fluid (ICF)** compartment. In an adult about 40% of body weight is intracellular fluid. *Intra-* is a prefix meaning within, or on the inside. This fluid compartment has the most protein in it.

   intracellular   The largest amount of body fluids is within the cells,
                          which is called the _____ compartment.

4. The fluid in each cell has its own unique composition, but the concentration of intracellular constituents is similar from one cell to another. For example, if you have three kinds of cookies, each cookie may contain different ingredients. Even though the cookies are not identical in composition, we call each of them a cookie, or three cookies. Although the intracellular fluid of individual cells differs in chemical composition, it is similar in concentration. Therefore, the intracellular fluid of all the different cells may be considered one large fluid compartment, even though it is contained in individual cells.

   similar   a. The concentration of constituents in each cell is (the
                             same, similar, different).
   composition   b. Each cell has its own chemical _____.

5. The second fluid compartment is known as the **extracellular fluid (ECF)** compartment and refers to all the fluid

outside the cells. In the adult approximately 20% of total body weight is extracellular fluid. The prefix *extra-* means outside. In school we participate in extracurricular activities. Extracurricular activities are pursuits that are not a part of the student's course of study but are still important for learning. Extracellular means outside the cell.

a. Fluid that is within the cell is called _____.

b. Fluid that is outside the cell is called _____.

intracellular
extracellular

6. The extracellular fluid outside the cell is divided into two smaller compartments: **interstitial** and **intravascular.**

Since *intra-* means within and *-vascular* means vessel, fluid that is within blood vessels is called _____.

intravascular

7. Although some of the extracellular fluid is within blood vessels (intravascular), the rest of the extracellular fluid is between the cells. Since this fluid is between the cells and blood vessels, it is called interstitial fluid.

Therefore extracellular fluid is divided into the following two parts:

a. _____

b. _____

intravascular
interstitial

8. If we divide all body fluid into only two groups and use the cell as our point of reference, then the fluids are either inside the cell or outside the cell.

The two main compartments for body fluids are:

a. _____

b. _____

intracellular
extracellular

9. We can divide the extracellular fluids further into two groups: those within the blood vessels and those between the cells.

The former group is called _____ and the latter _____.

intravascular
interstitial

10. Capillary walls and cell membranes separate the fluid compartments.

Fluid compartments are separated by _____ and _____.

capillary walls
cell membranes

11. Fluids outside the cells (intravascular and interstitial) are not static in content. They are constantly mixing together as they go through the capillary walls; therefore the capil-

lary wall serves as a blending chamber for extracellular fluid.

mixing   Extracellular fluids are (mixing, separate).

12. Label the body fluid compartments in the blanks provided at the left of Figure 1-1.

DISTRIBUTION OF BODY FLUIDS

The total body weight of an adult is 60% fluid (Figure 1-2); 40% of this fluid is inside the cells and 5% is within the blood vessels.

13. Newborn infants have a higher proportion of body weight that is fluid than do children and adults. At birth 75% to 80% of an infant's body weight is fluid. At approximately 2 years of age, the proportion of body weight that is fluid decreases.

75% to 80%   In infants the percentage of total body weight that is fluid is _____.

14. In infants the percentage of intracellular fluid is 40% of the body weight, the same as in young to middle-aged

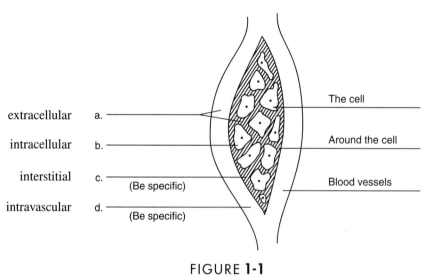

extracellular   a. ————————

intracellular   b. ————————

interstitial   c. ————————
                 (Be specific)

intravascular   d. ————————
                 (Be specific)

The cell

Around the cell

Blood vessels

FIGURE **1-1**
Body fluid compartments.

adults. However, in infants the extracellular fluid is approximately 35% of body weight, which is approximately 15% greater than the average adult.

The percentage of total body weight that is extracellular fluid in infants is approximately ___.   35%

15. With age, the total amount of water in the body diminishes. In the elderly the amount of intracellular fluid is reduced because of tissue loss. The percentage of total body weight that is fluid may be reduced to 45% to 50% in persons over age 65.

A person aged 65 is likely to have (45%, 60%, 75%) of body weight that is fluid.   45%

16. The percentage of total body water varies with age and the amount of body fat. Very little water is contained in fat

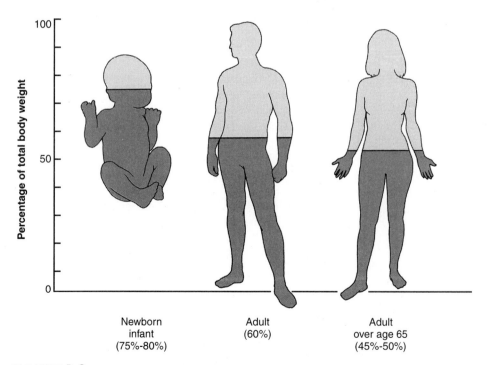

FIGURE 1-2

Proportion of body weight represented by fluid. Modified from Thibodeau GA, Patton KT: *Structure and function of the body,* ed 11, St Louis, 2000, Mosby.

(adipose) cells. Therefore persons with more body fat will have less total body water and be more susceptible to fluid imbalances.

less   A person who has more body fat will have (more, less) total body water than one who is lean.

17. The body must have fluid to continue its normal processes. Fluid output is regulated by the kidneys, through which the largest quantity of fluid is excreted. This excretion is known as sensible fluid loss. Other sources of sensible fluid loss are significant losses resulting from abnormal defecation, as with diarrhea, or from excessive amounts of perspiration or wound drainage. **Sensible fluid loss** is loss of fluid that can be measured. **Insensible fluid loss** refers to fluid loss that cannot be measured and is the result of normal respiration, perspiration, or defecation.

    a. An example of sensible fluid loss is fluid excreted

kidneys   through the _____.

insensible fluid loss   b. Daily fluid loss known as _____ is not measurable.

18. Fluid in the body is regulated by fluid intake, hormonal controls, and fluid output. Fluid intake is regulated by the ingestion of liquids, as the result of the thirst mechanism, and by the ingestion of food. The content of meats and vegetables is 60% to 97% water. Additional fluid is gained when food is broken down through the process of oxidation. (Water is one of the products of metabolism.) About 10 ml of water is released by the metabolism of each 100 calories of fat, carbohydrate, or protein.

    Two sources of fluid for the body are ingested liquids and the water in ingested foods.

    The third source of fluids for the body is that gained by

oxidation   the process of _____.

CONSTITUENTS OF BODY FLUIDS

ELECTROLYTES

19. When two or more atoms combine to form a substance, this is called a molecule. Atoms are composed of particles. The particles of an atom are the proton (positive

charge), electron (negative charge), and neutron (neutral). You can remember that the neutron is neutral because "neutron" and "neutral" begin with the same five letters. You can remember that the proton carries a positive charge because both "proton" and "positive" begin with the letter *p*. Finally, electron ends in the letter *n* and carries a negative charge. Electrical charges make cells function.

a. The electron of an atom carries a (positive, negative, neutral) charge.

    negative

b. The proton of an atom carries a (positive, negative, neutral) charge.

    positive

REMEMBER: An atom is the smallest particle of an element that still has the properties of the element.

---

20. The proton and neutron are in the nucleus, or center, of the atom.

    Therefore the nucleus is positively charged because it contains both the neutron, which is neutral, and the (proton, electron), which is positive.

    proton

21. Electrons carry negative charges and revolve around the nucleus. As long as the number of electrons in an atom is the same as the number of protons, there is no net charge on the atom (that is, it is neither positive nor negative). However, atoms may gain, lose, or share electrons and then no longer be neutral.

    If an atom either gains or loses electrons, it is no longer _____.

    neutral

22. When an atom carries an electrical charge because it has either gained or lost electrons and is no longer neutral, we call it an ion. An ion is an electrically charged atom or group of atoms.

    An atom that has an electrical charge is called a/an _____.

    ion

23. An ion may carry either a positive or a negative charge. When an ion carries a positive charge, it is called a **cation.**

    A cation is an ion with a (positive, negative) electrical charge.

    positive

REMEMBER: A cation is an ion that carries a positive electrical charge. A way to help you remember that cations are positive ions is to remember that "cation" has a "t," or plus sign (+), in it.

24. When an ion carries a negative electrical charge, it is called an **anion.**

negative   a. Anions carry a (positive, negative) electrical charge.

postive   b. Cations carry a (postive, negative) electrical charge.

25. **Anion gap** refers to the difference between the concentrations of serum cations and anions and can help determine the anion-cation balance. Identifying the gap that is present is useful in determining acid-base imbalances.

anion gap   The _____ detects acid-base imbalances.

26. **Electrolytes** are responsible for maintaining health and function in all body systems. An electrolyte is an element or compound that, when melted or dissolved in a solution, separates into ions and carries an electrical current.

health   Electrolytes help maintain _____ and _____.
function

27. Electrolytes are substances that dissociate (separate). Body fluids consist of water and dissolved substances. Some substances such as glucose, urea, and creatinine do not dissociate in a solution. That is, they do not separate from their complex form into simpler substances when they are in a solution.

do not   Glucose, urea, and creatinine (do, do not) dissociate when in solution.

28. Although some substances do not dissociate when in solution, other substances do dissociate. Electrolytes are electrically charged particles (ions) that dissociate, or separate, when in a solution. For example, when sodium chloride (NaCl) is in a solution, it dissociates, or separates, into two parts or elements.

Some   (Some, All) substances dissociate when in solution.

29. If we take an electrolyte such as sodium chloride (NaCl) and dissolve it in solution, it will dissociate into sodium (Na^+) and chloride (Cl^-).

Sodium is the cation because it carries a positive charge. Chloride carries a negative charge and is called

anion   the _____.

In solution, electrolytes dissociate into electrically charged ions. Therefore when an electrolyte is dissolved in water, it conducts an electrical current. We can demonstrate this by placing two electrodes in an electrolyte solution and connecting them to a bulb and battery. The dissociation of the electrolyte into charged atoms or ions will conduct an electrical current between the electrodes, and the bulb will light (Figure 1-3).

REMEMBER: Positive charges attract negative charges, whereas like charges repel.

30. The anion, the negatively charged ion, will migrate to the **anode,** which is the electrode with a positive charge.
    The anion $(-)$ will be attracted to the (positive, negative) electrode.   positive

31. Conversely, the negative electrode, which is called the **cathode,** will attract cations $(+)$ that have a positive charge.
    The cation is the (positive, negative) ion.   positive

    In summary, a negative ion (an anion) will be attracted to an electrode with a positive charge (an anode), and a positive ion (a cation) will be attracted to the cathode, an electrode with a negative charge.

32. If we put sodium chloride (NaCl) in a beaker to the level where the electrodes are immersed in the solution, what will happen to demonstrate that electricity has been conducted?
    a. The sodium (Na^+) will go to the (cathode, anode).   cathode
    b. The chloride (Cl^-) will go to the (cathode, anode).   anode

33. Electrolyte concentrations differ; however, the number of positive and negative charges within them balance to maintain **electroneutrality.**

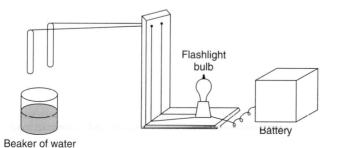

Flashlight
bulb

Battery

Beaker of water

FIGURE **1-3**
Example of action of electrolytes.

Balanced

(Balanced, Unbalanced) negatively charged and positively charged electrolytes are known as electroneutrality.

Measurement of Electrolytes

34. To study body fluids, we must have suitable units of measurement. To measure volume of fluids, we use the metric system and measure in liters (L) or milliliters (ml). A milliliter is one thousandth of a liter and is generally considered the same as a cubic centimeter (cc). Therefore we may say that a liter is equal to 1000 cc. In common usage, 1 cc is equal to 1 ml.

$\frac{1}{1000}$

A milliliter is what fraction of a liter? ($\frac{1}{10}$, $\frac{1}{100}$, $\frac{1}{1000}$).

We must have a unit of measure for the various electrolytes in body fluid. Because we are interested in the action of electrolytes (their ability to combine and form other compounds), the unit of measure must express their combining power (chemical activity). The combining power is a function of the number of ions. The weight of the ion has no relation to the chemical activity of the ion. Measuring electrolytes in units of weight such as milligrams per 100 ml does not tell us the chemical combining power of the electrolytes in solution (that is, how many cations, or positive ions, will be available to combine with anions, or negative ions). For example, if a hostess is having a party and wants couples of boys and girls, she does not invite 1000 pounds of boys for every 1000 pounds of girls. Their weight is not as important as the number of boys that will pair up with an equal number of girls.

REMEMBER: An equal number of cations and anions is necessary to maintain **homeostasis** (balance).

35. In measuring electrolytes, we are not concerned with how much they weigh (mg/100 ml). Instead, we want to know how many ions are available for chemical interaction.

activity

a. We want to know the chemical _____ of the electrolytes in solution.

ions

b. The chemical combining power of an electrolyte tells us how many ____ are available.

36. The unit of measure that expresses the combining activity of an electrolyte is the milliequivalent (mEq). An equivalent weight is the amount of one electrolyte that will displace or otherwise react with a given amount of hydrogen. Hydrogen is used as the yardstick or measure. To maintain acid-base balance, most electrolytes have to interact

with hydrogen ions: 1 mEq of any cation will always react chemically with 1 mEq of an anion, just as one boy reacts with one girl to make a couple.

   a. 100 mEq of cation will react chemically with ___ mEq of anion.

100

   b. 20 mEq of sodium (Na^+) will react with ___ mEq of chloride (Cl^-).

20

   c. If extracellular fluid has 155 mEq of cation, the number of milliequivalents of anion necessary for balance will be ___.

155

37. The fluid in each of the compartments (intracellular, interstitial, and intravascular) contains electrolytes. Each compartment has a particular composition of electrolytes, which differs from that of the other compartments. To function at optimal level, body cells must have fluids and electrolytes.

   _____ and _____ are necessary for body cells to function and maintain health.

Fluids
electrolytes

38. Electrolytes have different concentrations in both intracellular fluid (ICF) and extracellular fluid (ECF) and have different responsibilities to help maintain impulse transportation and cell membrane excitability. In the body, when potassium (K^+) is lost from the cell, the person becomes weak. If the potassium is not replaced, the person will die of myocardial necrosis and circulatory failure. (The heart muscle becomes soft, cannot pump blood, and dies as a result of the muscle and nerve fibers not being activated because of the lack of potassium within the cell.)

   Electrolytes (do, do not) play a major role in maintaining cellular excitability and impulse transportation.

do

A specific kind and amount of certain electrolytes must be available for normal cell function. In both ECF and ICF, even a small alteration in the concentration of electrolytes has the potential to cause significant health problems.

39. Whenever one electrolyte moves out of the cell, another will take its place. For example, if potassium is lost from the ICF, some other cation must replace it. Sodium, the most available cation in the ECF, moves into the cell. When electrolytes have to move from an area of lesser concentration (ICF) to an area of greater concentration (ECF) against a concentration gradient, it requires the use of **active transport.** An example of active transport is the

sodium-potassium pump. By exerting energy, **adenosine triphosphate (ATP)** sodium ions and potassium ions interchange to maintain homeostasis.

Active transport

_____ is the method in which the body moves electrolytes from an area of lesser concentration to an area of greater concentration.

✓ CONCEPT CHECK

Fluids and electrolytes are essential for health. The fluid compartments are intracellular and extracellular; the extracellular compartment includes interstitial and intravascular fluids. Body fluids contain water and electrolytes, the substances that dissociate in water into electrically charged particles called ions. Electrolytes are measured in milliequivalents, which express their combining power. The chemical combining power of an electrolyte is a measure of the number of ions. One milliequivalent of any cation will always react chemically with 1 mEq of any anion.

REMEMBER: Whenever an electrolyte moves out of a cell, another electrolyte moves in to take its place.

The number of cations and anions must be the same for homeostasis to exist. The use of physiologic pumps such as the sodium-potassium pump is a method of active transport that helps solutes move from areas of lesser to greater concentration.

✓ INFORMATION CHECK

1. The three fluid compartments in the body are:

intracellular   a. _____
intravascular   b. _____
interstitial   c. _____

substances that
dissociate in solution
into electrically
charged particles
called ions

2. Electrolytes are _____
_____
_____
_____
_____.

chemical combining
power

3. The number of ions available tells us the _____
_____ of an electrolyte.

the same number of

4. To achieve balance or equilibrium, we must have (more, fewer, the same number of) anions than (as) cations.

5. When one cation (for example, K^+) moves out of a cell, what happens? _____.

Another cation
moves in

6. ____ is the energy source of active transport.

ATP

NORMAL ELECTROLYTE COMPOSITION OF THE FLUID COMPARTMENTS

40. a. The major cation in both interstitial and intravascular fluid is _____.

sodium

   b. The total milliequivalents of anion are equal to the milliequivalents of _____.

cation

   c. The fluid compartment that has the most protein is the _____.

intracellular
compartment

   d. The chief cation in the intracellular fluid is _____ _____.

potassium (K^+)

   e. There is (more, less, a similar amount of) sodium in intracellular fluid than in intravascular fluid.

less

   f. The chief anion in interstitial and intravascular fluid is _____.

chloride (Cl)

MOVEMENT OF FLUID IN THE BODY

41. Fluids and **solutes** (the substances that are dissolved) move constantly throughout the body. This movement maintains homeostasis and balance. We have considered differences in composition of the intracellular, interstitial, and intravascular fluids. The difference in composition is partially caused by the nature of the barriers that separate the fluids. For example, cell membranes separate the interstitial fluid from the intravascular fluid. These barriers are selectively permeable, meaning they allow water and some solutes to pass through but not all of the solutes.

   a. Movement of water through the capillary wall is (unrestricted, restricted).

unrestricted

   b. (Some, All) solutes are allowed free passage through the walls of cells and capillaries.

Some

Diffusion

Water and solutes move through the walls of cells and capillaries in several ways. In effect, we have a mass transportation system to carry the traffic between the fluid compartments. These forces must carry the molecules of water, foods, gases, wastes, and many kinds of ions.

42. One process by which a solute (gas or substance) moves in solution is called **diffusion** (Figure 1-4). Diffusion is the movement of particles from an area of higher concen-

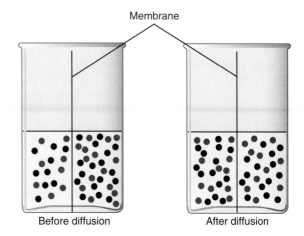

FIGURE 1-4
Diffusion across a semipermeable membrane. From Lewis SM, Heitkemper M, Dirksen S: *Medical-surgical nursing: assessment and management of clinical problems,* ed 5, St Louis, 2000, Mosby.

tration to an area of lower concentration and results in an equalization of solutes in both areas. For example, when you pour a small amount of cream into a cup of black coffee, the cream mixes or spreads through the whole cup of coffee and diffuses throughout (Christensen and Kockrow, 1998).

The process by which particles move from an area of higher concentration to an area of lower concentration is called _____.

diffusion

43. Diffusion is the process by which a solute may spread throughout a solution or solvent. A solute is the substance that is dissolved, a **solvent** is the solution in which the solute is dissolved.

solute

a. A substance that is dissolved is called the (solute, solvent).

b. The solution in which a solute is dissolved is called the (solute, solvent).

solvent

44. We have been discussing the diffusion of a solute throughout a solvent. Diffusion may also occur across a membrane if the membrane is permeable or allows free passage. When a membrane is permeable to a certain substance, that substance can go through the membrane freely. A permeable membrane will allow substances to pass through it without restriction. However, all the membranes in the body are selectively permeable, or semipermeable. A selectively permeable membrane will allow some solutes to pass through without restriction but will prevent other solutes from passing freely.

All the membranes in the body are (selectively, freely) permeable to some substances.

selectively

45. Diffusion occurs within fluid compartments and from one compartment to another if the barrier between the compartments is permeable to the diffusing substances. Diffusion is a very important process by which the solute and/or solvent may move freely from one fluid compartment to another. For example, the oxygen in the air we breathe enters the intravascular compartment and then goes into the cells by diffusion.

One process for the movement of fluids and (some, all) solutes is diffusion.

some

46. The type of diffusion we have described so far is called simple diffusion. Another way that a substance may diffuse across a membrane is by means of a carrier substance. An example of a carrier substance is insulin, which provides transport of glucose from the extracellular compartment into the cell. This is called facilitated diffusion. We might compare facilitated diffusion to a ski lift hauling skiers up a mountainside and then returning for more after dropping the first group at the top.

When a carrier substance is needed to transport another substance across a membrane, the process is called (simple, facilitated) diffusion.

facilitated

Osmosis

Osmosis involves the movement of a pure solvent, such as water, from an area of lower concentration to an area of higher concentration. This is a passive movement, and the process of osmosis stops when enough fluid has passed through the membrane and has resulted in an equal distribution of solutes/solvent. Equal concentration exists on both sides of the membrane. An example is the boiling of a hot dog. The concentration of molecules (solute) inside the hot dog is greater than the solvent (water). The skin of the hot dog acts as a semipermeable membrane and allows the water to pass into the hot dog freely. When the hot dog can no longer hold any more water, it ruptures (Christensen and Kockrow, 1998).

47. If a membrane is permeable to water but not to all the solutes present, it is a selective or semipermeable membrane. When the solvent or water moves across this membrane, we call the process osmosis.

The movement of fluid through a selectively permeable membrane is called _____.

osmosis

Semipermeable membrane

FIGURE **1-5**
Osmosis through a
semipermeable
membrane. From
Lewis SM,
Heitkemper M,
Dirksen S: *Medical-
surgical nursing:
assessment and
management of
clinical problems,* ed
5, St Louis, 2000,
Mosby.

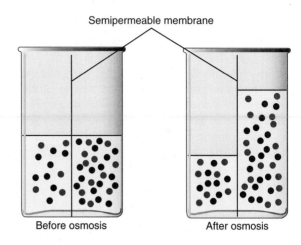

Before osmosis   After osmosis

48. Study Figure 1-5 and answer the following questions:
   a. Before osmosis the quantity of solution on both sides of the selectively permeable membrane is (different, the same).

the same

   b. After osmosis the quantity of solution on both sides of the membrane is (different, equal).

different

   c. (Solute, Solvent) has moved.

Solvent

   d. The reason the solvent moved is that the membrane will not allow the solute to go through; therefore the membrane is (permeable, selectively permeable).

selectively permeable

   e. After osmosis the concentration of salt solution on the two sides of the membrane is (the same, different).

the same

49. All normal living membranes are selectively permeable (that is, they do not allow all solutes free passage).
   a. The movement of water through such membranes is by the process of _____.

osmosis

   b. The result of osmosis is two solutions, separated by a membrane, that are (equal, unequal) in concentration.

equal

Filtration

50. **Filtration** is the process by which both solutes and solution move together in response to fluid pressure to create an equilibrium. Tissue perfusion is an example of filtration whereby water, nutrients, and waste products are exchanged at the capillary bed. This exchange occurs as a result of a difference in hydrostatic pressure between the capillaries and the tissue space.

   Solutes and solution move together to cause an equilibrium in a process known as _____.

filtration

51. When you have a more concentrated solution on one side of a selectively permeable membrane and a less concentrated solution on the other side, there is a pull called **osmotic pressure** that draws the water through the membrane to the more concentrated side, or the side with more solute.

    Osmotic pressure is the force that draws the water from a less concentrated solution through a selectively permeable membrane into a (less, equally, more) concentrated solution.

                                                                                                          more

52. The amount of osmotic pressure is determined by the relative number of particles of solute on the side of greater concentration. Therefore the greater the number of particles in the concentrated solution, the more pull there will be to move the water through the membrane.

    The force that pulls water across the membrane from the side of a less concentrated solution into a more concentrated solution is called _____.

                                                                                                  osmotic pressure

TYPES OF SOLUTIONS

Isotonic

53. When the solutions on both sides of a selectively permeable membrane have established equilibrium, or are equal in concentration, they are known as **isotonic.** *Iso-* is a combining form that means alike.

    When the solutions on both sides of a selectively permeable membrane are alike in concentration, they are

    _____.

                                                                                                        isotonic

54. One potential health problem is the inability to maintain adequate body fluids and proper chemical balance between the intracellular and the extracellular fluids. The movement of water through the cell membrane normally occurs so rapidly that any lack of osmotic balance is corrected within seconds. Therefore a state of osmotic equilibrium is maintained constantly when the body is functioning normally. When an extracellular fluid has the same concentration as the intracellular fluid, there is no net shift of fluid from outside the cell to inside the cell. When there is no imbalance and the solution is isotonic, it is considered to have no net fluid shift.

    Therefore, in this situation, the extracellular fluid is like, or _____ with, the intracellular fluid.

                                                                                                        isotonic

55. An example of an isotonic solution is 0.9% sodium chloride, which is referred to as isotonic saline solution or normal saline solution. This means that it is isotonic to human cells, and thus there will be very little osmosis.

0.9

An example of a solution that is isotonic to body cells is ___% sodium chloride.

56. When we say a solution is isotonic to another solution or to the intracellular fluid, we mean there (will be, will not be) movement of fluid from one side of the membrane to the other side by osmosis.

will not be

Hypotonic

57. When one solution contains a lower concentration of salt than another solution, we say it is **hypotonic.** *Hypo-* means less than ordinary. A hypotonic solution has less salt, or more water, than an isotonic solution.

less

A hypotonic solution has (more, less) salt than an isotonic solution.

58. A hypotonic solution is less concentrated than extracellular fluid and moves fluid from the bloodstream into the cells, causing them to enlarge. Distilled water is an example of a hypotonic solution because it does not have solutes in it. If we put distilled water on one side of a selectively permeable membrane and normal saline solution (0.9% sodium chloride) on the other side, water will move from the distilled water side to the normal saline side to make the solutions on both sides of the membrane more nearly equal in concentration. That is, both solutions will have an equal concentration of solutes to solution.

a hypotonic

Distilled water is an example of (a hypotonic, an isotonic) solution.

59. Because hypotonic solutions move fluid into the cells causing them to swell, patients with intracranial pressure should not be given hypotonic solutions. This type of solution will increase the fluid shift into the brain cells and result in a greater increase in cerebral swelling. Hypotonic solutions are also contraindicated in patients who have abnormal fluid shifts from the extracellular space into the intracellular space, such as occurs in patients with burns.

swell

Hypotonic solutions cause the cells to _____.

Hypertonic

60. **Hypertonic** solution pulls fluid from the cells, causing them to shrink and causing extracellular space to expand.

Dextrose 5% in half-normal saline is an example of a hypertonic solution.

Dextrose 5% in half-normal saline (is, is not) a hypertonic solution.   is

61. Hypertonic solutions must be used cautiously with patients who cannot tolerate additional extracellular fluids. Patients with renal or cardiac dysfunctions are at the greatest risk.

Hypertonic solution causes the cells to _____.   shrink

62. If either extreme fluid shift (swelling or shriveling of the cells) occurs in a person, death may result. Fluids and electrolytes must be kept in balance for optimal health.

Homeostasis results from fluid and electrolytes that are (balanced, unbalanced).   balanced

63. If the body loses more electrolytes than fluid, as occurs when a patient has diarrhea, the extracellular fluid will contain fewer electrolytes, or less solute, than the intracellular fluid. The concentration of solutes to solution is decreased. Fluids are pulled out of the cells into the bloodstream as an attempt to equalize the solute/solution ratio. If this process continues, the cells will continue to shrink and inhibit normal cellular function.

Therefore the fluid will be (pulled out of, pushed into)   pulled out of
the cells.

MEASUREMENT OF OSMOTIC PRESSURE

64. In an attempt to create an equilibrium, the osmotic pressure tries to proportionalize the number of particles per unit volume of solvent. The unit of measure of osmotic pressure is the osmole. Therefore the ability of solutes to cause osmosis and osmotic pressure is measured in terms of osmoles. In the body, the osmole is too large a unit for satisfactory use in expressing osmotic activity. The term milliosmole (mosm), which equals $1/1000$ osmole, is used to measure osmotic pressure in the body.

In the body the osmotic pressure is measured in
_____ (mosm).   milliosmoles

65. **Osmolality** means the number of osmotically active particles per kilogram of water.

The osmotic pull of all particles per kilogram of water
is called _____.   osmolality

66. A term closely related to osmolality is **osmolarity,** which refers to the number of osmoles per liter of solution, or the osmotic pressure of a solution.

osmolarity

The osmotic pull of all particles per liter of solution is called _____.

67. Osmolality is measured in milliosmoles per kilogram (mosm/kg) of water, and osmolarity is measured in milliosmoles per liter of solution (mosm/L). In the intravascular fluid, less of the weight is water, and the overall concentration of particles (solutes) is greater. The osmolality is greater than the osmolarity because of the smaller proportion of water.

greater than

The smaller proportion of water makes the osmolality (greater than, less than) the osmolarity.

68. Another way to think about osmolality is as the **specific gravity** of body fluids. Because specific gravity is the weight of the solution compared with an equal volume of distilled water, the osmolality of a solution can be estimated by the specific gravity. However, the osmolality of urine is a more concise measure of renal function than is the specific gravity. The kidneys respond to changes in osmolality rather than to changes in specific gravity. The normal osmolality of plasma is 280 to 294 mosm/kg.

280 to 294

The normal osmolality of plasma is _____ mosm/kg.

69. The osmolality of the extracellular fluid is determined mainly by the extracellular fluid concentration of sodium. Sodium is the most abundant extracellular cation and therefore provides 90% to 95% of the effective osmotic pressure of the extracellular fluid. Because of osmotic equilibrium, normally the extracellular fluid and the intracellular fluid have nearly the same osmolality.

sodium

The osmolality of the extracellular fluid is determined mainly by _____.

REMEMBER: Active transport system moves molecules or ions "uphill" against concentration, and osmotic pressure moves them "downhill" to areas of higher concentration.

70. Let's review. Diffusion and osmosis are passive processes (that is, they do not require energy from body cells). The natural tendency of molecules or ions is to

move from areas of higher concentration to areas of lower concentration. In diffusion, the molecules move to areas of lower solute concentration, and in osmosis the molecules move to areas with less solvent. Adenosine triphosphate (ATP) provides the energy needed for active transport. We have already discussed that an example of active transport is the sodium-potassium pump, which moves sodium to the outside of the cell and then returns potassium to the inside of the cell (Figure 1-6). However, the concentration of potassium is already much greater inside the cell than outside the cell. In addition to energy, a specific "carrier" molecule and a specific enzyme (ATPase) are required to promote active transport. Sodium, potassium, calcium, magnesium, some sugars, and amino acids use an active transport process to move from one compartment to another.

_____ and _____ are passive processes, but active transport requires energy and a specific enzyme.

Diffusion
osmosis

71. Solutes move by diffusion, and solvents by osmosis, from areas of high concentration to areas of low concentration.

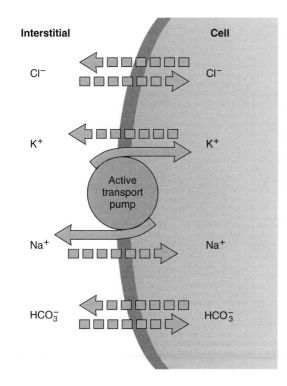

FIGURE 1-6
Sodium-potassium pump. From Beare PG, Myers JL: *Adult health nursing,* ed 3, St Louis, 1998, Mosby.

active transport

For substances to move in the opposite direction, an/a
_____ system is required.

Hydrostatic Pressure

72. We have considered the movement of fluids and electrolytes in the body by diffusion, osmosis, filtration, and active transport. Another type of movement of fluids and electrolytes is that resulting from **hydrostatic pressure** (Figure
1-7). Hydrostatic pressure is the force of fluid pressing outward against the vessel wall. When we relate hydrostatic
pressure to the blood, we are referring not only to the pressure of the weight of the fluid against the wall of the capillary but also to the force with which the blood is propelled
by each heartbeat. Because of the force of the blood pressure, the hydrostatic pressure at the arterial end of the capillary is approximately twice as great as it is at the venous end.

arterial

Hydrostatic pressure is greater at the (arterial, venous)
end of the capillary.

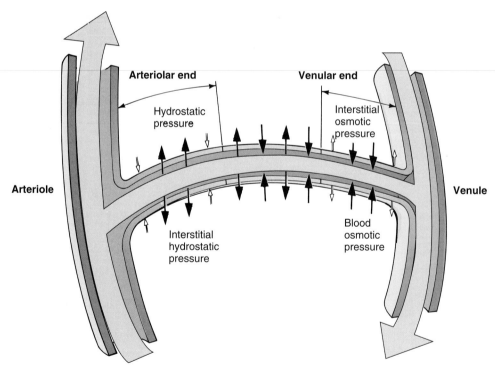

FIGURE **1-7**
Capillary hydrostatic and oncotic pressure. From Beare PG, Myers JL: *Adult health
nursing,* ed 3, St Louis, 1998, Mosby.

73. Hydrostatic pressure resulting from the process of filtration moves water and diffusible solutes from an area of higher pressure to an area of lower pressure.

    The process by which water and solutes pass through a membrane when the hydrostatic pressure is greater on one side of the membrane than on the other is called _____.   filtration

74. This tells us that hydrostatic pressure causes fluid and solutes, including nutrients, to be pushed out at the arterial end of the capillary.

    Hydrostatic pressure in the arterial end of the capillary results in fluid and solutes being _____.   pushed out

75. Because there is fluid in the interstitial space, there is also hydrostatic pressure in the interstitial space from the weight of the fluid. However, the hydrostatic pressure inside the arterial end of the capillary is greater (because of the heartbeat) than the interstitial hydrostatic pressure. Therefore fluid moves out of the capillary and into the interstitial space.

    Filtration is the movement of fluid through a selectively permeable membrane from an area with higher hydrostatic pressure to an area with ____ hydrostatic pressure.   lower

76. If the hydrostatic pressure at the arterial end of a capillary is 37 mm Hg and the hydrostatic pressure of the interstitial fluid is 1 mm Hg, the resultant difference, or pressure gradient, is 36 mm Hg and fluid is pushed out of the capillary.

    The difference in pressure gradient will cause fluid to move (out of, into) the arterial end of the capillary.   out of

77. However, osmotic pressure also affects the movement of fluid between the intravascular and interstitial compartments. The osmotic pressure caused by plasma colloids, or solutes, is called the **colloid osmotic pressure** or **oncotic pressure.**

    Oncotic pressure is the osmotic pressure that is caused by plasma _____.   colloids

REMEMBER: Osmosis is the movement of solvent molecules across a selectively permeable membrane, and osmotic pressure (or pull) is determined by the number of particles of solute on the concentrated side.

78. The protein content of intravascular fluid is different than that of interstitial fluid; intravascular fluid has more protein.

    Because intravascular fluid has more protein than interstitial fluid, the oncotic pressure, or pull, will tend to move fluids (into, out of) the capillary, or intravascular compartment.

into

79. Let us look at the result of hydrostatic pressure and oncotic pressure exerting force on the body fluids in the same place at the same time. When both pressures are at work in the arterial end of a capillary, hydrostatic pressure is pushing water and solutes out of the capillary, and the oncotic pressure is pulling water in. If blood has an oncotic pressure of 26 mm Hg and interstitial fluid has an oncotic pressure of 1 mm Hg, the oncotic **pressure gradient** will be 25 mm Hg, and the hydrostatic pressure gradient will be 36 mm Hg. This is a pressure difference of 11 mm Hg, which will result in a filtration action, or movement out of the arterial capillary (Table 1-1).

greater

a. Blood hydrostatic pressure is (greater, less) than interstitial fluid hydrostatic pressure.

greater

b. Blood osmotic pressure is (greater, less) than interstitial fluid osmotic pressure.

greater

c. Filtration force is (greater, less) than osmotic force.

out of

d. The result is that water and solutes move (into, out of) the capillary at the arterial end.

80. Now let us focus on the venous end of the capillary. We have already established that the hydrostatic pressure is

TABLE 1-1 ARTERIAL CAPILLARY PRESSURE	
ARTERIAL END OF CAPILLARY: HYDROSTATIC PRESSURE	
Blood hydrostatic pressure	37 mm Hg
Interstitial fluid hydrostatic pressure	− 1 mm Hg
Hydrostatic pressure gradient	36 mm Hg
ARTERIAL END OF CAPILLARY: OSMOTIC PRESSURE	
Blood osmotic (oncotic) pressure	26 mm Hg
Interstitial fluid osmotic pressure	− 1 mm Hg
Osmotic pressure gradient	25 mm Hg
Thus	
Filtration force = Hydrostatic pressure gradient	36 mm Hg
Osmotic force = Osmotic pressure gradient	− 25 mm Hg
Net filtration force	11 mm Hg

about half as great at the venous end of the capillary as it is at the arterial end. The pressures in the venous end of the capillary are described in Table 1-2.

a. At the venous end the blood hydrostatic pressure is (greater, less) than the osmotic force.   less

b. The result is that at the venous end of the capillary, water and solutes move (into, out of) the capillary.   into

c. Because of hydrostatic pressure and osmotic pressure, fluid and selected solutes move out of the capillary at the arterial end, whereas fluid and some solutes move into the capillary at the venous end (see Figure 1-7).

    Fluids and solutes enter the capillary at the venous end because of _____ pressure.   osmotic (oncotic)

81. About nine tenths of the fluid that filters out of the capillary at the arterial end is resorbed at the venous end. The other one tenth of the fluid is returned to the vascular system by the lymph channels. The lymphatics can carry proteins and large particles, which cannot be absorbed directly into the venous capillary, away from the tissue spaces. The permeability of the capillary wall varies in different parts of the body. For example, the capillaries in the liver allow protein to flow through their membranes, whereas the capillaries in the renal glomeruli normally do not allow protein through their walls.

    Capillary walls differ in their permeability to (solutes, solvents).   solutes

82. One example of a disturbance in the movement of fluids in the body occurs with patients who have congestive heart

TABLE 1-2 VENOUS CAPILLARY PRESSURE	
VENOUS END OF CAPILLARY: HYDROSTATIC PRESSURE	
Blood hydrostatic pressure	17 mm Hg
Interstitial fluid hydrostatic pressure	− 1 mm Hg
Hydrostatic pressure gradient	16 mm Hg
VENOUS END OF CAPILLARY: OSMOTIC PRESSURE	
Blood osmotic pressure	26 mm Hg
Interstitial fluid osmotic pressure	− 1 mm Hg
Osmotic pressure gradient	25 mm Hg
Thus	
Osmotic force	25 mm Hg
Filtration force	− 16 mm Hg
Net osmotic pressure	9 mm Hg

failure that develops into pulmonary edema. In this situation, the hydrostatic pressure in the lungs becomes severely increased. The hydrostatic pressure is increased so much that it overrides or exceeds the colloid osmotic pressure in the capillaries. The result is that large amounts of fluid from the capillaries move into the interstitial spaces in the lung.

out of

When the hydrostatic pressure in the capillaries exceeds the colloid osmotic pressure, fluid moves (into, out of) the capillaries into the interstitial space.

increase

83. Fluid entering the interstitial space will cause an (increase, decrease) in tissue congestion.

✓CONCEPT CHECK

Throughout the body the cell membranes and capillary walls are selectively permeable. Water and some solutes pass through the barriers freely, whereas other solutes require an active transport system.

Diffusion is the process by which a solute may spread throughout a solution. Molecules of a substance dissolved in a solvent spread by diffusion from an area of higher concentration to an area of lower concentration. When a carrier substance is needed to transport another substance across a membrane, the process is called facilitated diffusion. When molecules or ions move "uphill" against concentration and osmosis, energy from ATP and a carrier molecule, ATPase, are needed. This process is called active transport.

Osmosis is the movement of solvent molecules across a selectively permeable membrane to an area where there is a decreased concentration of solvent that is able to pass through the membrane. Because the solute particles cannot go through the membrane, the solvent moves to the area that has a lower solvent concentration. The result of osmosis is two solutions, separated by a membrane, that are more nearly equal in concentration of solutes.

Osmotic pressure is the force that draws the solvent from a solution with more solvent molecules through a selectively permeable membrane to a solution with fewer solvent molecules. The amount of osmotic pressure is determined by the relative number of particles of solute on the side of greater concentration. When the solutions on each side of a selectively permeable membrane are equal in concentration, they are isotonic. A hypotonic solution has less solute than an isotonic solution, and a hypertonic solution contains more solute than an isotonic solution. If the selectively permeable membrane will allow the solvent to pass through but will not allow the solute through freely, the solvent will move to the side of greater solute concentration. If an ion is to move through a membrane from an area of low concentration to an area of high concentration, an active transport system is necessary.

Osmolality refers to the number of osmotically active particles per kilogram of water. In the body, osmotic pressure is measured in milliosmoles. The normal osmolality of plasma is 280 to 294 mosm/kg.

Hydrostatic pressure is the force of the fluid pressing outward against some surface. When there is a difference in the hydrostatic pressure on two sides of a membrane, water and diffusible solutes move out of the solution that has the higher hydrostatic pressure. This process is called filtration. At the arterial end of the capillary, the hydrostatic pressure is greater than the osmotic pressure. Therefore fluid and diffusible solutes move out of the capillary. At the venous end the osmotic pressure, or pull, is greater than the hydrostatic pressure, and fluids and some solutes move into the capillary. The excess fluid and solutes remaining in the interstitial space are returned to the intravascular compartment by the lymph channels.

INFORMATION CHECK

1. The process by which particles spread in all directions through a solution is called _____.

diffusion

2. The movement of fluid through a selectively permeable membrane is called _____.

osmosis

3. The force that draws solvent from a solution with more solvent through a selectively permeable membrane into a solution with less solvent is called _____.

osmotic pressure

4. When the solutions on both sides of a selectively permeable membrane are alike in concentration, they are _____.

isotonic

5. If cells are placed in a hypotonic solution, they will _____ and may _____.

swell
burst

6. The process by which water and solutes pass in unison through a membrane when the hydrostatic pressure is greater on one side of the membrane than on the other is called _____.

filtration

7. Water and some solutes move out of the capillary at the arterial end because the hydrostatic pressure gradient is greater
osmotic   than the _____ pressure gradient.

8. At the venous end of a capillary, water and some solutes move into the capillary because the filtration force is less
osmotic (oncotic)   than the _____ force.

NORMAL REGULATION MECHANISM BY WHICH WATER AND ELECTROLYTES ENTER AND LEAVE THE BODY

84. Normally fluids enter the body through three sources: oral liquids, water in foods, and water formed by oxidation of foods. Electrolytes are present in both foods and liquids. With a normal diet, an excess of essential electrolytes is taken in, and the unused electrolytes are excreted.
     Water is taken into the body through the following three sources:

oral liquids   a. _____
water in foods   b. _____
oxidation of foods c. _____

85. The typical amount of fluid intake over a 24-hour period for an adult is about 2200 to 2700 ml/day. Table 1-3 describes the breakdown of an adult's intake.
     The largest quantity of water is taken into the body as
oral (ingested) liquids   _____.

86. Generally, the amount of liquids that infants ingest in a 24-hour period is approximately equal to the amount of urine they excrete in that same 24 hours; the water they gain in a day through ingestion of food sources and oxidation of food is approximately the same amount as the water they excrete through feces and evaporation in a 24-hour period (Wong, 1999).
     Table 1-4 describes the daily maintenance fluid re-

TABLE 1-3	ADULT AVERAGE DAILY FLUID GAINS AND LOSSES		
Fluid Gains	**(ml)**	**Fluid Loss Location**	**(ml)**
Ingested liquids	1100-1400	Kidneys	1200-1500
Water in foods	800-1000	Skin	500-600
Water from oxidation	300	Lungs	400
		Gastrointestinal	100-200
TOTAL GAINS	2200-2700	TOTAL LOSSES	2200-2700

From Potter PA, Perry AG: *Fundamentals of nursing*, ed 5, St Louis, 2001, Mosby.

quirements per body weight. Infants and young children have greater fluid needs and are more susceptible to fluctuations in fluid balance. The relationship of total body weight and the immaturity of the regulation systems makes the need for homeostasis greater.

a. Infants need (more, less) fluid per kilogram of body weight than do adults.

more

b. At 6 months of age, an infant who weighs 9 kg may require (100, 200, 400) ml of fluid per kilogram of body weight over a 24-hour period.

100

c. Infants and young children are (more likely, less likely) to be vulnerable to fluid alterations.

more likely

87. An adult requires approximately 2200 to 2700 ml of fluid over a 24-hour period; a 20-lb (9.1 kg) infant requires 100 ml of fluid per kg of body weight over a 24-hour period.

The fluid needs of an adult are (more than, less than, the same as) those of an infant.

less than

We previously discussed insensible and sensible fluid loss in general. Let us now review these mechanisms in greater detail. Fluids leave the body by several routes. These are detailed in Table 1-5.

88. Insensible fluid loss accounts for lost fluid that generally cannot be seen or measured. One way this fluid is lost is through the skin. Water is lost through the skin of an adult

TABLE 1-4 DAILY MAINTENANCE FLUID REQUIREMENTS	
Body Weight (kg)	Amount of Fluid/Day
1-10	100 ml/kg
11-20	1000 ml plus 50 ml/kg for each kg >10 kg
>20	1500 ml plus 20 ml/kg for each kg >20 kg

From Wong DL, et al: *Whaley and Wong's nursing care of infants and children,* ed 6, St Louis, 1999, Mosby.

TABLE 1-5 INSENSIBLE AND SENSIBLE FLUID LOSSES	
Source	Amount
INSENSIBLE FLUID LOSSES	
Skin	500-600 ml
Lungs	400 ml
SENSIBLE FLUID LOSSES	
Urine	1200-1500 ml
Intestines	100-200 ml

From Potter PA, Perry AG: *Fundamentals of nursing,* ed 5, St Louis, 2001, Mosby.

by diffusion in the amount of 500 to 600 ml/day. Refer to Table 1-5. The amount of water lost by diffusion through the skin is obligatory (that is, it will be lost regardless of intake). We are not aware of losing water through the skin in this way; therefore it is called insensible perspiration. In other words, it cannot be measured.

The amount of water lost through the skin by diffusion is about _____ ml/day.

500-600

89. Another insensible loss of fluid is through expired air, which is saturated with water vapor. The amount of water lost from the lungs will vary with the rate and depth of respirations. The average amount of water lost from the lungs in an adult is about 400 ml/day. The water lost from the lungs and through the skin by diffusion is called insensible loss because we are unaware of losing that water.

In an adult the total average amount of water that we say is an insensible loss via the skin is (100, 400, 700) ml/day.

400

90. Sensible fluid loss can be measured. Large quantities of fluid are secreted into the gastrointestinal tract, but almost all of this fluid is resorbed. The average amount of water lost in the feces of an adult is 100 to 200 ml/day.

The normal amount of water lost through the feces of an adult is _____ ml/day.

100-200

91. The gastrointestinal (GI) system plays a significant role in fluid balance. About 3 L to 6 L of electrolyte-containing liquid moves into the GI tract and then returns again to the extracellular fluid. This is a significant amount of liquid, so we can understand why any abnormal loss of GI secretions, such as occurs with diarrhea, is important and how it can lead to critical changes in the maintenance of fluid balance.

An abnormal loss of secretions from the GI tract is (serious, unimportant).

serious

92. The organs that play a major role in regulating fluid and electrolyte balance are the kidneys. More than any other organ in the body, normal kidneys can adjust the amount of water and electrolytes leaving the body. The quantity of fluid excreted by the kidneys is determined by the amount of water ingested and the amount of waste or solutes excreted. The usual quantity of urine output for an adult is approximately 1200 to 1500 ml/day. However, this will vary greatly depending on fluid intake, amount of

perspiration, and several other factors. Urine output can be measured and is considered to be a sensible fluid loss.

a. The major organs that regulate fluid and electrolyte balance are the _____.   kidneys

b. The usual quantity of urine output for an adult is _____ ml/day.   1200-1500

93. An infant's kidneys are immature and unable to concentrate or dilute urine. Therefore an infant requires more water and has difficulty conserving body water.

An infant requires (more, less, the same amount of)   more
water per kilogram of body weight than does an adult.

REMEMBER: The amount of urine excreted in a 24-hour period depends on fluid intake, state of health, and age (see Table 1-4). As long as all organs are functioning normally, the body is able to maintain balance.

CONTROLS FOR MAINTAINING FLUID AND ELECTROLYTE BALANCE

If a person is to remain healthy, the volume, concentration, and composition of fluids and electrolytes must be maintained within narrow limits. This is an extremely complex task when we consider the billions of cells in the body constantly pouring the products of chemical reactions into the extracellular fluid and withdrawing from it substances needed for specific cellular activities. What we take into the body as food and fluid contains a wide variety of materials. Some food contains electrolytes at a concentration far in excess of levels permissible in body fluid.

94. The volume of liquids we drink might drown us were there no mechanisms for maintaining a constant volume of body fluid. These needs for maintaining balance, or homeostasis, are multiplied when the body is fighting disease.

The volume, concentration, and composition of body fluids must be _____.   maintained

95. Homeostasis is the goal of the relatively stable internal environment. The composition of the internal environment may vary from tissue to tissue because of differences in cell activity and metabolism. Yet, because of the movement of substances between the compartments (by means of osmosis, diffusion, filtration, and active transport), a relative consistency is maintained. We recognize, then, that the internal environment is not static but is instead dynamic.

Homeostasis implies (stagnation, variation within   variation within limits
limits).

The maintenance of homeostasis depends on a variety of processes. Substances that the cells need must be available in adequate quantity. Some of the substances required by the cell are oxygen, water, and a variety of nutrients including calories, tissue-building materials, and electrolytes.

96. The intake, storage, and elimination of the substances must be maintained within safe limits. In health, the body is able to respond to disturbances in levels of fluids and electrolytes so as to prevent or repair damage.

    Health and balance is achieved when fluid and electrolytes maintain a _____ state.

    homeostatic

97. Thirst, the conscious desire for water, is one of the major factors that determines fluid intake. The osmoreceptors in the hypothalamus are cells that are stimulated by an increase in the osmotic pressure of body fluids to initiate thirst. After eating potato chips you become thirsty because the salt on the chips increases the osmotic pressure of body fluids.

    a. In a healthy person one of the major factors that regulates fluid intake is _____.

    thirst

    b. When the osmotic pressure of the body fluids increases, the _____ in the hypothalamus are stimulated to initiate thirst.

    osmoreceptors

98. Thirst is also stimulated by a decrease in the extracellular fluid volume. This is another way in which the body attempts to regain balance—by increasing the intake of fluids.

    A decrease in the volume of extracellular fluid will stimulate _____.

    thirst

99. Fluid intake is also regulated by the dryness of the mouth as a result of decreased salivary secretion. A dry mouth does stimulate thirst but is not necessarily the result of decreased fluid intake. For instance an individual who has been given the drug Atropine, a drug that prevents salivation, will become thirsty even though there is no deficit in fluid volume.

    A decrease in salivation (will, will not) stimulate thirst.

    will

100. In a healthy person, thirst is stimulated by the following factors:

    a. (Increased, Decreased) osmotic pressure

    Increased

    b. (Increased, Decreased) extracellular fluid volume

    Decreased

    c. (Dry, Moist) mucous membranes in the mouth

    Dry

101. It is important that nurses realize that an individual such as an infant, a young child, or an older adult who is unable to communicate thirst is at risk. Although thirst is a major stimulus for acquiring fluid intake, individuals who are not able to assume the responsibility of obtaining fluids on their own should be offered plenty of opportunities for hydration.

An infant, a young child, or an adult who cannot communicate the sensation of thirst (is, is not) at risk for alteration in fluid balance.

is

102. Homeostasis of the volume of water in the body is maintained or restored by adjusting the output to the intake. The kidneys assume the major responsibility for maintaining balance of both fluids and electrolytes and do so by controlling output. They are master chemists and remove waste materials or excessive substances from the extracellular fluid. The kidneys excrete varying amounts of water and resorb or release sodium, potassium, bicarbonate, and hydrogen ions to regulate intracellular and extracellular concentrations within normal limits.

Normally functioning kidneys are essential in regulating _____ and _____ balance.

fluid
electrolyte

103. Healthy kidneys excrete and resorb varying amounts of water and other substances to regulate intracellular and extracellular concentrations. The volume of urine is regulated primarily by hormones from the posterior lobe of the pituitary gland (antidiuretic hormone) and the adrenal cortex (aldosterone). Being influenced by these hormones, the kidneys help regulate the total volume of extracellular fluids, the ratio of water to solutes (concentration), and the specific quantity of the different electrolytes (composition).

_____ and _____ hormones help the kidneys regulate urine output.

Antidiuretic
aldosterone

104. When the extracellular fluid volume becomes too high, the blood volume, or intravascular volume, is increased. Therefore the venous return to the heart is increased, which then increases the cardiac output. This results in an increased arterial pressure. The increased arterial pressure resulting from the increased fluid volume causes the kidneys to excrete the excess fluid.

When the volume of extracellular fluid is too high, the kidneys respond by excreting (more, less) urine.

more

105. Normally the interstitial fluid volume is regulated so as to keep the interstitial fluid spaces filled. However, when this balance is not possible because of an underlying disease process, the interstitial spaces can become expanded with excess fluid. Excess fluid in the interstitial spaces is called **edema.**

interstitial
    Edema is the result of increased fluid in the _____ _____ spaces.

106. When the extracellular fluid volume is decreased because of increased loss or inadequate intake, the kidneys respond by retaining more fluid, so the extracellular fluid volume is returned to more nearly normal. However, if the extracellular fluid volume deficit is too great, the complex mechanisms affecting the kidney may not be enough to correct the imbalance, and treatment becomes necessary.

less
    When the extracellular fluid volume is decreased, the kidneys respond by excreting (more, less) urine.

107. Helping to maintain an adequate fluid balance is the function of two hormonal systems. One of these is the aldosterone system. **Aldosterone** is a hormone secreted by the adrenal cortex that regulates the extracellular volume by affecting the renal control of sodium and potassium.

aldosterone
    The hormone from the adrenal cortex that affects extracellular fluid volume is _____.

108. Aldosterone, released by the adrenal cortex, acts on the distal portion of the renal tubules to increase the reabsorption (saving) of sodium, chloride, and water and the secretion of potassium and hydrogen. Generally with sodium retention there is water retention and the regulation of extracellular volume.

more
    a. When there is an increased production of aldosterone, the kidneys retain (more, less) sodium, chloride, and water.

loss
    b. At the same time, an increased production of aldosterone causes a (loss, gain) of potassium.

109. Aldosterone production is a complex and not completely understood mechanism. In a healthy person an increased production of aldosterone occurs when there is low fluid volume, low blood sodium, and high blood potassium. This process is a normal compensatory mechanism that is a continual process throughout the lifespan. When an individual's compensatory mechanism no longer regulates

fluid volume adequately, that individual's health or (homeostasis) can become compromised.

Although the excretion or retention of sodium, chloride, potassium, and water occurs as a function of the kidneys, one of the hormones that affects this regulation is

_____.

aldosterone

110. In a healthy person the production of aldosterone is controlled to maintain a balance of fluids and electrolytes in the body. If, because of disease, the adrenal glands become overactive and secrete more aldosterone than needed for homeostasis, a serious imbalance may occur. Various diseases of the adrenal glands result in overproduction of aldosterone. Cushing's syndrome is one disease in which the adrenal glands are overactive.

You would expect the symptoms of Cushing's syndrome to be the result of excretion of _____ and retention of _____, _____, and ____.

potassium
sodium, chloride
water

111. If the adrenal glands become extremely underactive, the excretion of potassium will be decreased; that is, more potassium will be retained in the body. Also, the levels of sodium, chloride, and water will decrease because these ions are lost from the body in the urine. In persons who have various diseases such as AIDS or metastatic cancer or who have had an adrenalectomy, the adrenal glands are hypoactive.

A person whose adrenal glands are very underactive will excrete a (large, normal, small) amount of urine.

large

112. We have looked briefly at some ways the kidneys are influenced by the hormone aldosterone to control the volume of extracellular fluid. Another hormone that affects extracellular fluid is the **antidiuretic hormone (ADH).** ADH is secreted by the posterior pituitary gland. Its name explains its action, *anti-* meaning against and *-diuretic* meaning increased secretion of urine. We could say that ADH is the water conservation hormone.

An increase in the production of ADH will lead to an increase in (urine production, urine saving).

urine saving

REMEMBER: The H in the abbreviation ADH should recall the word "hold" to help you remember that an increase in ADH will lead to an increase on the HOLD of urine output.

113. ADH regulates the osmotic pressure of extracellular fluid by regulating the amount of water resorbed from the blood by the renal tubules and makes them more permeable to water. This, in turn, allows the water to return to the circulating system and leads to the dilution of blood and an increase in osmolarity.

ADH (antidiuretic hormone)

The hormone that is secreted by the posterior pituitary gland and that acts to conserve fluid is _____ _____.

114. The ADH mechanism is complex, but the results of the action of ADH can be easily summarized. If there is an increased production of ADH, there will be increased amounts of water resorbed by the kidney through osmosis. The urine volume will be decreased, but the concentration will be increased.

decreased

The result of increased production of ADH is (increased, decreased) volume of urine.

115. The usual stimulus that causes production of ADH is an increase in the osmotic pressure of the extracellular fluids. ADH stimulates a retention of fluid to correct this increase in osmotic pressure. For example, if a large amount of hypertonic glucose solution is infused into the body, the osmotic pressure of the extracellular fluid will be increased. This will stimulate the production of more ADH, so more fluid will be retained and the osmotic pressure of the extracellular fluid will be returned to normal.

osmotic

ADH production is regulated by changes in _____ pressure.

Renin, an enzyme that is secreted by the kidneys, responds to a decrease in renal perfusion as a result of a decreased extracellular volume. Renin produces **angiotensin I,** which acts to cause some vasoconstriction. Angiotensin I is reduced by an enzyme that converts angiotensin I into **angiotensin II,** which creates selective vasoconstriction and causes a redirection of blood flow to the kidneys that will improve renal perfusion. Angiotensin II also stimulates the release of aldosterone when the serum sodium concentration is low.

116. For health to be maintained, the volume, concentration, and composition of body fluids and electrolytes must be kept within narrow limits. The regulation of these factors depends on intake and excretion.

Regulation of the loss of water and electrolytes depends

primarily on the kidneys, which are affected by the hormones _____ and _____ and by the enzyme _____.

ADH
aldosterone
renin

117. There may be an imbalance in the volume, concentration, or composition of body fluids. Any change in any one of these three can result in alteration of a fluid balance and homeostasis.

Fluid balance is evaluated based on _____, _____ and _____.

volume
concentration
composition

EXAMPLES OF FLUID AND ELECTROLYTE IMBALANCE

We have discussed three types of body fluid imbalance: volume, concentration, and composition. In the text below we discuss each imbalance separately, but we must remember that most patients will have a combination of imbalances.

EXTRACELLULAR FLUID VOLUME IMBALANCE

118. Extracellular fluid volume imbalance may be a deficit in the volume of fluid without significant changes in the electrolyte concentration. A deficit can be caused by an abrupt reduction in fluid intake, such as when a patient is to take "nothing by mouth" (NPO) per doctor's orders or when a person is not ingesting food or fluid by mouth in preparation for being given an anesthetic or when the person is trying to avoid stimulating the GI tract.

_____ imbalance is the result of a decrease in fluid intake without any significant changes in the electrolyte concentration.

Fluid volume

119. The signs and/or symptoms the nurse should look for in assessing fluid volume deficit include depression of the central nervous system (evidenced by reduced energy or stupor), depression of GI activity with or without vomiting (evidenced by a decrease in bowel sounds), reduced blood volume (evidenced by a decrease in blood pressure), an increase in heart rate (as a compensatory mechanism to override the decreased blood volume), dry mucous membranes, and increased body temperature.

The signs and symptoms related to a fluid volume deficit correlate to those associated with a depressed

_____.

central nervous
system

120. In the treatment of extracellular fluid volume deficit without a significant change in the electrolyte concentration,

fluids with electrolytes resembling the electrolytes in normal extracellular fluid are given. If the patient cannot be given fluids orally, the physician will order fluids to be given parenterally (for example, by intravenous infusion).

A patient who is taking nothing by mouth will have a
fluids   deficit of _____, unless they are replaced parenterally.

EXTRACELLULAR FLUID CONCENTRATION IMBALANCE

121. A deficit in electrolyte concentration can occur in a patient who has a nasogastric tube in the stomach and loses both fluids and the electrolytes sodium and potassium that are drained by suction. In the treatment of such a patient, fluids containing electrolytes will be ordered by the physician to restore the normal balance of both fluids and electrolytes.

electrolytes

Fluids ordered to supplement a loss of extracellular fluid concentration should contain _____.

122. Subsequently, if the nasogastric tube is irrigated with water, even more electrolytes will be washed out. Therefore the tube must be irrigated only enough to keep it patent, or open. An isotonic solution such as normal saline (0.9% sodium chloride) should be used for irrigation.

sodium
potassium

A patient who has a nasogastric tube connected to suction will lose water and especially the electrolytes, _____ and _____.

EXTRACELLULAR FLUID COMPOSITION IMBALANCE

123. An example of an imbalance in the composition of electrolytes in body fluid is a deficit in potassium. A deficit in potassium can occur in infants who have diarrhea, in adults who have ulcerative colitis (a disease marked by numerous bouts of watery diarrhea bowel movements), in burn patients who are healing (because potassium shifts back into the intracellular compartment), and in others with conditions such as diaphoresis and vomiting. Normally, when potassium (in very small quantities) moves out of the cell, sodium replaces it. This activity causes an electrochemical impulse to be transmitted along the nerve and muscle fibers. If potassium is not available in the cell, activating impulses are not transmitted to the muscles or nerves.

potassium

The lack of the electrolyte _____ alters neuromuscular impulses.

124. The nurse should assess for neuromuscular depression that may vary from loss of muscle tone to coma.

   The degree of variation in neuromuscular depression associated with the loss of potassium is considered (small, large).

large

125. Subsequently, there is depression of the GI tract with paralytic ileus (absence of peristalsis), and the electrocardiogram will show changes. When the potassium deficit becomes severe, marked cardiac conduction abnormalities occur.

   a. Activating impulses (are not, are) transmitted to the muscles or nerves when potassium is not available in the cell.

are not

   b. The major cation in the intracellular fluid is _____.

potassium

> **REMEMBER:** Under no circumstances can potassium chloride (KCl) be given IV push. A direct IV infusion of KCl is *fatal.*

126. When potassium has been lost from the cell because of the depletion of potassium in the extracellular fluid, several days of therapy may be needed to restore the depleted intracellular stores. Potassium may be given orally or parenterally. The exchange of fluids between the intravascular and interstitial spaces occurs rapidly through the capillary. By comparison, the rate of exchange of electrolytes across the cell membrane is slow.

   a. If potassium is depleted in the extracellular fluid to the extent that the intracellular potassium becomes low, (minutes, hours, days) of therapy may be required to restore the intracellular potassium level.

days

   b. Potassium administered as a direct IV push is ____.

fatal

127. Since potassium is one of the ions necessary for the transmission of impulses to muscles and nerves, a severe deficit in potassium that is not corrected can be serious. Death may result from weakness of the respiratory muscles and myocardial failure.

   Death may result from weakness of the respiratory muscles and myocardial failure when there is (a deficit, an excess) of potassium.

a deficit

> **REMEMBER:** Almost any patient who has an imbalance of fluids or electrolytes will have a combination of imbalances.

✓ CONCEPT CHECK

The volume, concentration, and composition of body fluids must remain nearly constant. The kidneys play a major role in controlling all types of balance in fluids and electrolytes. The adrenal glands, through secretion of aldosterone, also aid in controlling extracellular fluid volume by regulating the amount of sodium resorbed by the kidneys. ADH from the pituitary gland regulates the osmotic pressure of extracellular fluid by regulating the amount of water resorbed by the kidneys. When one of the substances (fluids or electrolytes) is deficient, it must be replaced by either normal intake of food and water or by medical therapy, such as intravenous infusions and/or medication. When there is an excess of fluids or electrolytes, therapy is directed toward helping the body to eliminate the excess.

✓ INFORMATION CHECK

excess fluid in interstitial spaces
1. Edema is the result of _____.

2. The organs primarily responsible for the regulation of volume, concentration, and composition of body fluids are the

kidneys _____.

sodium
potassium
3. A person who has gastric suction or has had prolonged vomiting will have a deficit of water, _____, and _____.

a combination
4. The type of imbalance most likely to occur in a patient is _____.

● KEY POINTS

1. Body fluids are distributed in functional compartments that are intracellular and extracellular.

2. The extracellular compartment includes interstitial and intravascular fluids.

3. Body fluids contain water and electrolytes.

4. Electrolytes are measured in milliequivalents (mEq), and for normal balance the milliequivalents of cations and anions must be equal.

5. Diffusion, osmosis, filtration, active transport, and hydrostatic pressure are methods that promote the movement of fluids between the compartments.

6. An imbalance may occur in volume, concentration, or composition of the fluid.

7. For health, fluids and electrolytes must be in balance.

8. Antidiuretic hormone (ADH) regulates the amount of water resorbed by the kidneys.

9. Aldosterone regulates the amount of sodium resorbed by the kidneys.

10. Renin, in response to a decrease in renal perfusion, produces angiotensin I to create some vasoconstriction. Angiotensin I is converted to angiotensin II, which causes a more selective vasoconstriction and redirects blood flow to the kidneys, thereby increasing renal perfusion.

?CRITICAL THINKING QUESTIONS

1. Describe why an infant is more likely to develop a fluid imbalance than a school-aged child. _____
_____

A higher percentage of an infant's body weight is fluid

2. Explain why a client with previous health problems is at greater risk for developing fluid and electrolyte imbalances.
_____
_____
_____
_____
_____

Body fluid and acid-base balance is the result of healthy, normally functioning cells

3. What will happen when a hypertonic IV solution is administered to a patient? _____
_____
_____

ECF becomes diluted and cells become rehydrated

4. In what scenario should hypertonic solution administration be given cautiously? _____
_____
_____
_____
_____
_____
_____
_____
_____

Clients with heart disease and renal failure should be treated cautiously because hypertonic IV solutions pull fluids into the vascular space and cause an increase in vascular volume

Another cation moves in

5. When one cation (for example, potassium) moves out of the cell, what happens? _____ _____

ATP as an energy source moves sodium to the outside of the cell and then returns potassium to the inside of the cell

6. What role does ATP play in maintaining the balance of the sodium-potassium pump? _____ _____ _____ _____ _____

Potassium must **NEVER** be administered as an IV push medication; it must be diluted in IV solution and administered over a specific period of time

7. Describe the appropriate method of administering potassium by the parenteral route. _____ _____ _____ _____ _____ _____ _____ _____

An insensible loss or gain is generally not perceived by an individual; a sensible loss or gain, on the other hand, is measurable, as in the case of urine output

8. What is the difference between insensible and sensible fluid losses and gains? _____ _____ _____ _____ _____ _____ _____

Children are more susceptible to fluid loss than adults and, secondly, they are more susceptible to fluid overload—related problems during hydration

9. Describe the fluid needs of a child versus those of an adult. _____ _____ _____ _____ _____ _____ _____ _____ _____

FLUID VOLUME IMBALANCE

INTRODUCTION

Disturbance of body fluids usually results in some type of illness, either at the local or systemic level. The nurse must be aware of the various body fluid disturbances, how they develop, and what characterizes them. The ability to return the patient to a state of health is the goal of fluid management.

You have completed the program that presents the normal distribution and constituents of body fluids, as well as the controls for maintaining fluid and electrolyte balance. As a nurse you share with the physician the responsibility for making observations that will serve as a basis for decisions regarding the fluid and electrolyte status of the patient. The nurse is available to make assessments not only of the patient's intake and output but also of the symptoms and signs relative to fluid needs. The nurse has the added responsibility of ensuring that those patients who are unable to understand and communicate their need of adequate fluid intake, such as infants, young children, and some impaired adults, are offered fluids at appropriate intervals. Nurses must be keenly aware of a patient's fluid output to be able to assist the patient in maintaining a fluid balance homeostasis.

Fluid volume imbalance is more likely to occur and more likely to be severe in infants, young children, and the elderly than it is in older children or young to middle-aged adults. The greater need for fluids that infants have combined with their larger body surface area relative to their weight contributes to their potential for fluid imbalance. Infants also have higher metabolic rates, resulting in greater heat production and greater insensible fluid loss, in addition to a greater need for fluid excretion. Kidney function is immature at birth, so infants have a limited capacity for concentrating or diluting urine. In the elderly, homeostasis is fragile; their bodies experience a decline in the ability to compensate for imbalances effectively, in addition to having decreased total body water as compared to younger adults. With increasing age, the sensation of thirst is reduced and the ability to concentrate urine declines, which may result from poor renal response to the antidiuretic hormone (ADH) and may also be related to a decreased number of nephrons in the kidney. All of these variations in body compo-

KEY TERMS

colloid solutions
crystalloid solutions
dehydration
diabetes insipidus
fluid volume
overload
hematocrit
hemoconcentrated
plasma
hemoglobin
hypertonic
dehydration
hypotonic
dehydration
hypovolemic
isotonic dehydration
third spacing

sition and function make assessing for fluid imbalance in infants, young children, and the elderly especially important.

128. You may recall that the chief sources of body fluid intake when a person is healthy are:

ingestion of liquids   a. _____

water in food solids   b. _____

metabolism (water   c. _____
from oxidation)

129. Normally fluid losses occur through the gastrointestinal

kidneys   (GI) tract, the lungs, the skin, and the _____.

FLUID VOLUME DEFICIT

130. The body loses water constantly throughout life. A deficit in the body's fluid volume may occur for two reasons: it may simply be the result of an inadequate intake, or it may result because output is increased over the intake. Water alone may be lost, but electrolytes can be lost as well. In fluid volume deficit (dehydration), water and electrolytes can be lost together (isotonic volume deficit), electrolytes can be lost at a greater rate than fluid (hypotonic volume deficit), or fluid can be lost at a greater rate than electrolytes (hypertonic volume deficit). With each of these volume deficits, fluid management is necessary to return the patient to a state of balance.

Water deficit may occur for the following reasons:

inadequate intake   a. _____

excessive output   b. _____

131. Whenever the loss of water from the body exceeds the intake, water is extracted from the extracellular fluid compartment. The result is that the remaining extracellular fluid becomes hypertonic in relation to the intracellular fluid. Hence the fluid is shifted out of the cells into the extracellular compartment in an attempt to compensate.

According to the law of osmosis, water can be ex-

out of   pected to move (out of, into) the cell.

dehydration or   132. This results in cellular _____.
crenation

133. Because the extracellular fluid becomes hypertonic, the osmotic pressure is increased. The increase in osmotic pressure in the extracellular fluid stimulates the sensation of thirst. This is problematic for infants, young children, impaired adults, or elderly persons because they are likely not to have the ability to communicate thirst or they may

have an impaired sense of thirst and therefore may not
drink enough fluid.

    a. When water is available and the person is able to in-
gest and absorb it, a fluid volume deficit can be corrected by _____.

                                                                 drinking water

    b. Individuals who are at risk for an altered thirst com-
pensatory mechanism are _____, _____,
_____, and _____.

                                                                               infants
young children
impaired adults

134. When the osmotic pressure of the cells becomes relatively
less than that of the extracellular water, the posterior pituitary gland secretes more ADH, which leads to a decrease
in urinary output for the purpose of conservation.

                                                                          the elderly

    In a fluid volume deficit, as a result of the decreased
blood volume flowing through the kidneys and the increased secretion of ADH, normally functioning kidneys
will excrete (more, less) urine.

                                                                          less

> ***REMEMBER:*** When there is a fluid volume deficit, the volume of extracellular water
> is decreased. This causes the adrenal glands to secrete aldosterone, which causes a
> retention of sodium and thus water.

LABORATORY FINDINGS

135. No single laboratory test results in a diagnosis of fluid
volume deficit. Along with clinical manifestations, a patient with either isotonic or hypotonic dehydration will
have a **hemoconcentrated plasma.** That is, the **hematocrit** (the proportion of erythrocytes to blood plasma) and
hemoglobin (the percentage of oxygen-carrying iron)
will be elevated. A normal hematocrit is 35% to 45% for
women and 40% to 50% for men. A normal hematocrit
for infants is 28% to 42% and 35% to 45% for children.
The normal hemoglobin for women is 11.7 to 16.1 g/dl,
12.6 to 17.4 g/dl for men, 9.0 to 14.0 g/dl for infants, and
11.5 to 15.5 g/dl for children.

    a. The normal hematocrit for a newborn is (higher,
lower) than any other age group (Table 2-1).

                                                                          higher

    b. In a person with a fluid volume deficit, the hemoglobin
will be (higher, lower) than normal for others in that
age group.

                                                                          higher

136. The severity and type of dehydration will determine the
loss of electrolytes in the extracellular fluid (ECF). In
many cases electrolyte loss can be the result of an under-

TABLE 2-1	HEMATOCRIT IN CHILDREN	
	Age	**Hematocrit**
	Newborn (1-3 days)	44% to 75%
	Infant (2 months)	28% to 42%
	Child (6-12 yrs)	35% to 45%

From Wong DL, et al: *Whaley & Wong's nursing care of infants and children*, ed 6, St Louis, 1999, Mosby.

lying health problem or the result of a side effect of a medication (as with diuretic therapy). Generally when a patient has a fluid volume deficit, the patient also has an increase in the ratio of sodium and other electrolytes in the plasma.

deficit

A (deficit, excess) in fluid volume generally is related to an increase in sodium and other electrolytes in the plasma.

137. Healthy kidneys adapt to a fluid volume deficit by excreting a small volume of concentrated urine. The normal specific gravity of urine is 1.010 to 1.025. Along with an increase in specific gravity related to an increase in concentration, the patient's urine will be darker in color and have an odor. When an adult has adequate kidney function, an output of less than 500 to 800 ml in 24 hours is indicative of inadequate water intake. Both infants and the elderly have a decreased ability to concentrate urine. Therefore they are more likely to develop a fluid volume deficit.

Which of the following test results would indicate fluid volume deficit?

_____ a. Serum sodium 140 mEq

b   _____ b. Hematocrit 55% in a 3-year-old child

c   _____ c. Specific gravity of urine 1.040

_____ d. Serum chloride 103 mEq

138. Which of the following individuals is most likely to be unable to concentrate urine?

a   _____ a. 3-month-old Jill

_____ b. 10-year-old Angie

_____ c. 40-year-old Mr. Brown

d   _____ d. 92-year-old Mrs. Graham

SIGNS AND SYMPTOMS

139. In assessing a patient, the nurse will look for signs and symptoms of fluid volume deficit. Thirst is the earliest

symptom of water deficit, and this occurs when there is an increased plasma osmolarity or a decreasing plasma volume.

A(n) _____ or a(n) _____ _____ is responsible for initiating the thirst mechanism.

increase in plasma osmolarity

decrease in plasma volume

140. As ECF is lost, the osmotic pressure of the remaining fluid is increased, and water moves from the cells into the extracellular compartment. Therefore the intracellular fluid (ICF) volume is decreased. Apparently, the hypothalamus is sensitive to the decreased ICF volume and produces the sensation of thirst. Patients who are apathetic, confused, or very ill are at risk for developing a water deficit. The sense of thirst may be impaired in infants, in persons with cerebral injury, and in the elderly.

The thirst mechanism is initiated by the _____.

hypothalamus

141. Other patients at risk for fluid losses are those with an elevated temperature because they lose an excessive amount of water from the lungs. The patient with a tracheostomy is likely to have an accelerated pulmonary water loss because the dead air fraction of the tidal volume is reduced. An excessive loss of water may occur in patients with burns because of the shift and remobilization of fluids they experience. For these patients and all patients who have the potential to become fluid volume depleted, the nurse should provide adequate amounts of water given in a palatable form.

The following patients are likely to need additional fluid intake:

a. _____

b. _____

infants

patients with cerebral injury

c. _____

d. _____

the elderly

apathetic and confused patients

e. _____

f. _____

patients with elevated temperature

tracheostomy patients

g. _____

burn patients

142. In an alert, competent person the earliest symptom of a fluid volume deficit is _____.

thirst

143. A fluid volume deficit is also likely to occur when a person has difficulty swallowing or has no gag reflex or when a patient is comatose. It is interesting to remember that such patients have an intact fluid and electrolyte balance. Their potential for fluid volume deficit is related to the inability to swallow fluids or to their unconscious state.

inability

The (inability, ability) to ingest fluids can result in a fluid volume deficit. Hence although patients may have an intact fluid balance, they are at risk for an alteration in their fluid status if they are incapable of ingesting fluids.

144. Patients with **diabetes insipidus** (a disorder marked by an extensive loss of water) who cannot concentrate water because of a lack of ADH and patients with an intrinsic kidney disease who may have an inability to conserve water are at risk for fluid volume deficits. The nurse should be alert to other signs and symptoms (an increase of urinary output, changes in mucous membranes or weight) consistent with fluid volume deficit, especially when thirst is not indicated by the patient.

increase
change

The potential for fluid volume deficit occurs when a patient exhibits an _____ in urinary output or a _____ in mucous membranes or weight.

145. When the water deficit is significant, skin and mucous membranes and weight may provide signs that indicate fluid volume status. A weight change of 1 pound indicates a fluid loss of 500 cc of fluid. Dry, cracked mucous membranes also are indicative of an inadequate fluid intake. (However, a dry and fissured tongue also may occur in a person who is a mouth breather or who is receiving oxygen by mask.) The skin may be flushed, and perspiration may be decreased. An adult with fluid volume deficit has little saliva, and the urine output is less than 500 ml in 24 hours. Although thirst is a symptom of fluid volume deficit in alert persons, the nurse should also be aware of signs of fluid volume deficit.

Which of the following signs may indicate fluid deficit?

_____ a. Moist, clean mucous membranes

b
_____ b. Urine output of 400 ml in 24 hours in an adult

_____ c. Cool, moist skin

d
_____ d. Dry, fissured tongue

146. In addition to the signs discussed previously, the patient
     with a fluid volume deficit may have marked physical
     weakness and exhibit confusion or delirium and may have
     a decrease in blood pressure and an increase in heart rate.
       Signs of severe water deficit include the following:
     a. _____   weakness
     b. _____   delirium
     c. _____   confusion
     d. _____   decreased blood
                                                           pressure
     e. _____   increased heart rate

TYPES OF FLUID VOLUME DEFICITS

Dehydration

147. **Dehydration** (fluid volume deficit) is one of the most com-
     mon body fluid disturbances in infants and children. When-
     ever output of fluid exceeds intake, dehydration occurs.
       The most common body fluid disturbance in infants is

     _____.   dehydration

> **REMEMBER:** Infants ingest and excrete a greater amount of fluid per kilogram of
> body weight than do older children or adults.

148. Some infants are born with a congenital abnormality that
     can affect body fluid volume. However, fluid volume
     deficit in infants typically results from immaturity and is
     frequently caused by gastroenteritis. Because an infant
     has a relatively greater body surface area compared to an
     adult in relation to body weight, large quantities of fluid
     can be lost through the skin.
     a. An infant has a relatively (smaller, greater) body sur-   greater
        face area in relation to weight than does an adult.
     b. Infants can lose a significant quantity of fluid through
        the ____.   skin

149. Three types of dehydration are isotonic, hypotonic, and hy-
     pertonic. In **isotonic dehydration** the loss of fluid and elec-
     trolytes is approximately balanced in proportion. Most of
     the loss is sustained by the extracellular compartment. Iso-
     tonic dehydration is the most common type of dehydration.
       In isotonic dehydration there is a loss of both elec-
     trolytes and ____.   fluid

150. Another type of dehydration is **hypotonic dehydration,** in which electrolyte deficit is greater than fluid deficit. Because the extracellular fluid is hypotonic, it moves into the intracellular space. Therefore the extracellular fluid volume becomes even less. The physical signs and symptoms of deficit tend to be more severe with hypotonic dehydration.

greater

In hypotonic dehydration the deficit of electrolytes is (less, greater) than the deficit of fluid.

151. The third type of dehydration is **hypertonic dehydration,** in which the deficit of fluid is greater than the deficit of electrolytes. Because fluid then shifts out of the intracellular space and into the extracellular space, the physical signs and symptoms of fluid volume deficit are not as apparent, but neurologic disturbances become evident.

into

a. In hypertonic dehydration fluid shifts (into, out of) the extracellular compartment.

less

b. In hypertonic dehydration the physical signs and symptoms of fluid volume deficit are (more, less) apparent than in hypotonic dehydration.

152. Because infants and small children are unable to describe their symptoms, the nurse must be observant to detect changes (Table 2-2). In isotonic and hypotonic dehydration, skin turgor is lost. However, in hypertonic dehydration the skin will feel firm (as a result of the fluid shift into the extracellular compartment).

lost

In isotonic dehydration skin turgor is (lost, firm).

153. The mucous membranes become dry when a patient has isotonic dehydration. The eyeballs appear sunken and soft. In an infant, the fontanel becomes sunken or depressed (Figure 2-1), and the pulse and respirations become rapid.

Which of the following may indicate an isotonic dehydration?

_____ a. Moist mucous membranes

b   _____ b. Sunken eyeballs

c   _____ c. Depressed fontanel

_____ d. Slow pulse and respirations

154. Other significant changes that occur with isotonic dehydration include a decrease in weight from the pre-illness weight, a decrease in urinary output, and an increase in

TABLE 2-2 PHYSICAL SIGNS OF DEHYDRATION			
	Isotonic (Loss of Water and Salt)	Hypotonic (Loss of Salt in Excess of Water)	Hypertonic (Loss of Water in Excess of Salt)
Skin			
Color	Gray	Gray	Gray
Temperature	Cold	Cold	Cold or hot
Turgor	Poor	Very poor	Fair
Feel	Dry	Clammy	Thickened, doughy
Mucous membranes	Dry	Slightly moist	Parched
Tearing and salivation	Absent	Absent	Absent
Eyeball	Sunken	Sunken	Sunken and soft
Fontanel	Sunken	Sunken	Sunken
Body temperature	Subnormal or elevated	Subnormal or elevated	Subnormal or elevated
Pulse	Rapid	Very rapid	Moderately rapid
Respirations	Rapid	Rapid	Rapid
Behavior	Irritable to lethargic	Lethargic to comatose; convulsions	Marked lethargy with extreme hyperirritability on stimulation

Modified from Wong DL, et al: *Whaley & Wong's nursing care of infants and children,* ed 6, St Louis, 1999, Mosby.

specific gravity. It is important that any or all of these signs or symptoms be recorded and reported.

a. With a fluid volume deficit, the infant's weight will
_____.   decrease

b. The specific gravity of the urine will _____.   increase

155. In the elderly, dehydration is the most common cause of fluid and electrolyte disturbance. This is partially because of the decrease in total body water, the reduced sense of thirst, and a reduction in urinary concentrating ability that occurs with increasing age.

a. One cause for dehydration in the elderly is (increased, decreased) thirst.   decreased

b. With increasing age, the kidneys become (less, more) able to concentrate urine.   less

156. With the aging process it is generally normal for the tissue turgor to decrease with the loss of subcutaneous fat, causing wrinkling of the skin. This should not be interpreted as a sign of dehydration.

Wrinkled skin in the elderly (is, is not) always a sign of dehydration.   is not

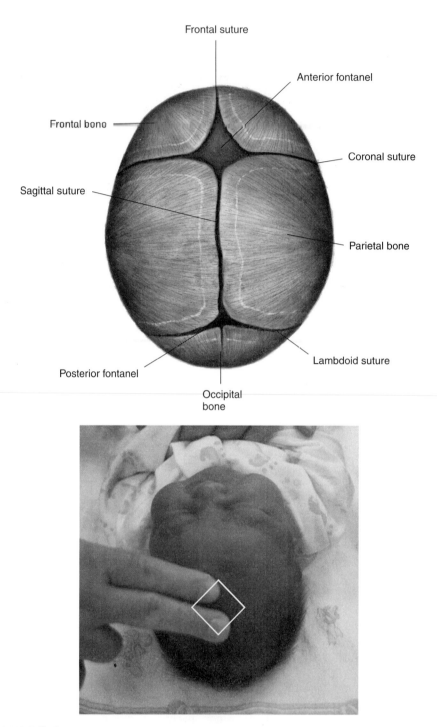

FIGURE 2-1

A, Location of sutures and fontanels. **B,** Palpating anterior fontanel. From Wong DL, et al: *Whaley & Wong's nursing care of infants and children,* ed 6, St Louis, 1999, Mosby.

157. With most cases of fluid volume deficit, the nurse moni-
tors the patient to detect signs and/or symptoms and col-
laborates with the physician on treatment. Collaborative
management therapy focuses on prevention of further
losses and replacement of fluids, either orally if the deficit
is mild to moderate or intravenously if the loss is moderate to severe or the individual cannot ingest fluids orally.

   Monitoring a patient at risk for a fluid volume deficit
(is, is not) an appropriate nursing activity.   is

158. As part of the management therapy, the nurse should plan
for and then provide a variety of fluids to the patient at appropriate time intervals. Nurses must realize that just of-
fering fluids may not be sufficient for some patients. The
nurse may need to assist the patient with fluid intake.

   A variety of fluids given at intervals (should, should not)   should
be offered to all patients who are not on fluid restriction.

159. An excessive overload of fluid, caused either by a very
large volume of fluid being given intravenously or by a
person drinking a large volume of water, will result in a
significant increase in urinary output. If urinary output
exceeds intake, an individual may experience a fluid volume deficit.

   Although not a common cause, an imbalance of fluid
_____ can be produced by giving excessive amounts   volume
of ingested or intravenously administered water.

✓CONCEPT CHECK

Whenever loss of water from the body exceeds intake, water is
extracted from the ECF compartment. Because the extracellular
fluid becomes hypertonic, the osmotic pressure is increased and
thirst results. The nurse must be alert for patient conditions in
which development of water deficit could occur and observe
and report any signs and/or symptoms. Marked physical weakness and confusion are signs of severe water deficit.

✓INFORMATION CHECK

1. When the volume of fluid is decreased, the concentration of
sodium and other electrolytes in the plasma will be
_____.   increased

2. When there is a deficit in the fluid volume, the hematocrit
and hemoglobin will be _____.   elevated

3. The following patients are likely to need additional fluid:

confused patients   a. _____

very ill patients   b. _____

patients with elevated   c. _____
temperature

patients with a   d. _____
tracheostomy

burn patients   e. _____

infants   f. _____

patients with cerebral   g. _____
injury

4. Signs of fluid deficit include the following:

dry, cracked mucous   a. _____
membranes

flushed skin   b. _____

decreased urine   c. _____
output

5. Signs of fluid deficit in an infant include the following:

eyeballs sunken and   a. _____
soft

fontanel sunken or   b. _____
depressed

rapid pulse and   c. _____
respirations

weight loss   d. _____

FLUID REQUIREMENTS

160. Table 1-3 shows the average fluid requirements for adults. In a person with normally functioning kidneys, the volume of fluid intake should be approximately the same as the volume of fluid output.

The average volume of urine per 24 hours for an adult

1200 to 1500   is approximately _____ ml.

161. An average adult requires approximately 1100 to 1400 ml of fluids per day. In some instances, such as when a person has an increase in body temperature or has increased perspiration, additional water may be necessary.

increase   An increase in perspiration may require a(n) _____ in fluid replacement.

162. Fluid loss created by perspiration is variable but can reach a maximal rate of about 2 L/hour with exertion or when a

person is in a hot environment. It is important to understand also that for each increased degree Celsius of body temperature there will be an increase in insensible fluid loss of about 10% (Ignatavicius et al, 1999). Under both of these circumstances, the increased loss of fluid causes an increased need for fluid replacement. If the loss is significant and/or goes untreated, an individual's intake will not be balanced with output.

Therefore a person with an elevated temperature will need a(n) (increased, decreased) amount of water.   increased

163. Other causes for increased loss of fluid include vomiting, diarrhea, gastrointestinal drainage, burn exudate, internal pooling (ascites), significant wound exudate, or a side effect or therapeutic effect resulting from a medication.

When assessing a patient for a fluid volume deficit, it (is, is not) important to obtain a history of health problems and medication regimens.   is

164. Fluid requirements for infants are listed in Table 1-4. As with children, fluid needs for infants are based on their weight and age. For example, an infant who weighs about 10 kg, approximately 20 lbs, would require 100 ml/kg per day or 1000 ml/day. Additionally, as the infant matures, there is a change in his/her basal metabolic rate (BMR increases with growth) and body surface area (BSA changes with age, the newborn has a 2 to 5 times greater BSA than does a child), and, as the kidneys mature, there is an increase in efficiency to excrete urine (Table 2-3).

Fluid requirements for infants change based on their:

a. _____   weight
b. _____   age
c. _____   BMR

TABLE 2-3	URINE OUTPUT BY AGE	
	Age Group	Output in ml/24 hr
	Newborn	50-350
	Infant	350-500
	Child	500-1000
	Adolescent	700-1400
	Thereafter:	
	Adult male	800-1800
	Adult female	600-1600

From Wong DL, Hess CS: *Wong and Whaley's clinical manual of pediatric nursing,* ed 5, St Louis, 2000, Mosby.

BSA	d. _____
maturity of kidneys	e. _____

It is important that the nurse understand that subsequent to these normal physiologic changes, determination of appropriate fluid replacement for an infant or child also must take into consideration any present health alterations and illnesses, such as gastroenteritis or burns or an increase in environmental temperature or body temperature.

165. An infant or child with an elevated temperature will have an increase in his/her insensible water loss by approximately 7 ml/kg/24 hours for each degree Celsius (C) rise in temperature above 37.2° C .

A child who has a temperature of 38.2° C and weighs 20 kg will experience an increase in his/her insensible fluid loss in 24 hours by _____.

7 ml/kg

166. It is important for the nurse to understand that for the infant and child, an increase in perspiration will proportionately increase the need for added fluids to maintain fluid balance.

A child who has an elevated body temperature and is perspiring will need (an increased, a decreased) amount of fluid.

an increased

167. The elderly are another population vulnerable to dehydration. As a person ages, a decrease in the total amount of body fluid occurs, and therefore his/her need for liquid intake is slightly less than that of younger adults. An elderly client's kidneys are less able to concentrate urine, have fewer functioning nephrons, and have a decrease in the glomerular filtration rate. However, their output will remain high, which will require an equal amount of intake.

Even though total body water is less in the elderly, their intake and output (does, does not) change significantly from that in younger adults.

does not

TREATMENT

168. Water can only be given orally. For many adults and children, a water deficit can be prevented by providing adequate amounts of water in a clean, palatable form. The most satisfactory way for a patient to ingest water is to drink from a glass or cup while in the sitting position. For alert patients, providing more drinking water may be all

that is necessary to increase fluid intake. Some patients, especially infants, young children, and elderly persons, may require assistance. For patients who must remain supine, their heads should be turned to the side, if possible, to make it easier for them to drink. Patients should be given an explanation of how much fluid intake is desirable and why.

The most satisfactory way to provide fluid intake for children and adults is _____ _____.

by having them drink from a glass while sitting up

FLUIDS BY INFUSION

169. Water can be given orally, except when fluids by mouth are contraindicated. When fluids cannot be given orally, the parenteral route (IV) may be necessary. The volume to be infused generally is based on the patient's signs and symptoms and weight, and the type of solution to be infused is based on the type of fluid volume deficit the patient is experiencing. Subsequently the rate of the IV infusion depends on the degree of the dehydration and the presence of any pre-existing cardiac, pulmonary, or renal health problems (Ignatavicius et al, 1999).

The amount of IV solution that should be given for fluid replacement (is, is not) based on the patient's signs and symptoms, weight, and the type of deficit.

is

170. The physician determines which fluids will be given parenterally. Sometimes **colloid solutions** are used in the treatment of severe fluid volume deficit or shock. Colloid solutions are composed of a continuous medium, throughout which small particles (1 to 1000 nm in size) that do not separate out are distributed. A nanometer (nm) is equal to 1 billionth of a meter. These particles are not capable of passing through a semipermeable membrane. Examples of colloid solutions include whole blood, plasma, packed red blood cells, and dextran.

Colloid solutions (do, do not) pass through a semipermeable membrane.

do not

171. Since colloids do not pass through a semipermeable membrane, they are retained in the vascular system. Colloids increase the osmotic (oncotic) pressure in the vascular system. Therefore more fluid is drawn into the vascular system, and the circulating blood volume increases.

Colloids cause fluid to be (drawn into, pushed out of) the vascular space.

drawn into

172. Usually crystalloids (noncolloidal substances) are used to treat a fluid volume deficit. A crystalloid is a substance in a solution that can be diffused through a semipermeable membrane. Table 2-4 shows a list of **crystalloid solutions.** Crystalloids can be divided into the following categories: isotonic, hypotonic, and hypertonic. Isotonic solutions have the same effective osmolality as body fluids, whereas hypotonic solutions have an effective osmolality less than body fluids and hypertonic solutions have an effective osmolality greater than body fluids (Horne and others, 1997). The type of crystalloid solution given intravenously most often is an isotonic solution.

Crystalloid   _____ solutions can be diffused through a semipermeable membrane.

173. One example of an isotonic solution that could be given intravenously is dextrose 5% in water. Dextrose is metabolized quickly, which leaves the water free to be distributed evenly through all fluid compartments (Horne and others, 1997).

isotonic   Dextrose 5% in water is a(n) (hypotonic, isotonic, hypertonic) solution.

174. The decision of whether to use a hypotonic or hypertonic solution is based on the patient's fluid and electrolyte imbalance. For example, a hypotonic solution of 0.45%

TABLE 2-4 INTRAVENOUS SOLUTIONS	
Solution	**Type**
DEXTROSE IN WATER SOLUTIONS	
Dextrose 5% in water	Isotonic
Dextrose 10% in water	Hypertonic
SALINE SOLUTIONS	
0.45% sodium chloride	Hypotonic
0.9% sodium chloride	Isotonic
3%-5% sodium chloride	Hypertonic
DEXTROSE IN SALINE SOLUTIONS	
Dextrose 5% in 0.9% sodium chloride	Hypertonic
Dextrose 5% in 0.45% sodium chloride	Hypertonic
MULTIPLE ELECTROLYTES SOLUTIONS	
Lactated Ringer's	Isotonic
Dextrose 5% in lactated Ringer's	Hypertonic

Modified from Potter PA, Perry AG: *Fundamentals of nursing,* ed 5, St Louis, 2001, Mosby.

sodium chloride (½ normal saline) would be used to treat a hypertonic dehydration.

The use of a hypotonic solution will result in rehydration of the cells.

Hypertonic dehydration is best treated by a (hypotonic, hypertonic) IV solution.   hypotonic

---

REMEMBER: In a hypertonic dehydration the fluid shift causes fluid to move from the ICF to the ECF and results in shrinkage and dehydration of cells.

---

175. All IV therapy should be given according to the prescribed physician's order and given with great care. Evaluation of serum laboratory studies, along with the patient's history and physical exam, usually helps the physician determine what type of fluid volume deficit the patient is experiencing. Overloading the patient with fluid by failing to follow the prescribed order exactly regarding the volume, type, and rate of fluid to be administered can result in serious health problems. For example, a hypertonic solution such as dextrose 5% in sodium chloride has the potential to cause pulmonary edema, particularly in patients with heart or renal health problems, because of the increase of fluid in the vascular space.

IV solution (should, should not) be administered   should
carefully.

176. The potential danger to the patient is increased when fluids are given intravenously because fluids go immediately into the systemic circulation. Although the physician is responsible for the prescription of the amount, character, and route of administration of the patient's intake, the nurse is usually responsible for the administration of the fluids. Therefore the nurse must know how to give fluids in a safe and effective manner. The nurse must also be sure that the patient gets the correct solution in the proper amount and at the rate prescribed. The nurse must also see that sterility of the solution and the equipment is maintained.

The nurse is responsible for (prescription, admin-   administration
istration) of fluids.

177. When giving any medication, the nurse checks to verify that the right drug in the proper dose, at the prescribed time, and by the correct method of administration is given to the right patient.

To give intravenous fluids safely and effectively, the nurse should identify the patient and see that he or she gets the right ____ in the proper ____ at the ____ prescribed.

drug, dose, time

178. All patients should be observed at regular intervals when fluids are given parenterally. The nurse should not rely on assistant personnel to check the rate of infusion. Observation is especially important in patients whose homeostatic or compensatory mechanisms are inadequate or have been challenged as a result of the patient's physical immaturity (as with an infant or small child) or underlying health problems. Patients with limited renal function and/or cardiac reserve are in danger of pulmonary edema or congestive heart failure. Very young patients, as well as older patients, are less able to tolerate large volumes of fluid given rapidly. The nurse is responsible for the safe administration of fluids.

Pulmonary edema or congestive heart failure is more likely to occur in patients with limited ____ function and/or ____ reserve.

renal
cardiac

179. The nurse should be alert to symptoms that indicate **fluid volume overload,** such as occur with congestive heart failure. If the patient becomes short of breath or has dyspnea (difficult breathing), the flow rate should be decreased and the physician notified. An increase in the respiratory rate, coughing, or the development of cyanosis suggests a fluid overloading of the patient's circulation and movement of fluid into the alveoli of the lungs.

Pulmonary edema and congestive heart failure are likely to be accompanied by the following symptoms:

shortness of breath   a. _____

dyspnea   b. _____

increased respiratory   c. _____
rate

coughing   d. _____

cyanosis   e. _____

180. The rate of administration of intravenous fluids depends on the need for fluids and the nature of the fluid being given. The physician will prescribe exactly how fast the fluid should be given intravenously. The rate of flow will affect the safety and the state of comfort of the patient. Fluids given over a 12- to 24-hour period contribute more to the patient's comfort and to fluid and electrolyte balance than do fluids administered over a shorter period

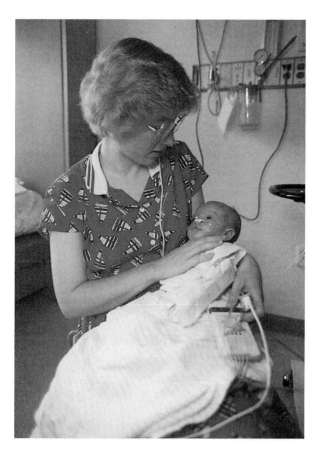

FIGURE **2-2**
Intravenous infusion, as well as other equipment, does not prevent an infant from being picked up and cuddled. From Wong DL, et al: *Whaley & Wong's nursing care of infants and children,* ed 6, St Louis, 1999, Mosby.

(Figure 2-2). The rate of flow affects the value of the fluids to the patient.

Fluids given over a period of (4 to 12, 12 to 24) hours will be safest and most effective.

12 to 24

181. The rate of administration varies with the condition of the patient and the nature of the fluid. The patient must be observed frequently during administration. Shortness of breath or dyspnea may indicate that the rate is too rapid. The nurse must be alert to the patient's urinary output in relation to the fluid intake and must observe and report signs of too rapid a rate of administration.

A patient who is receiving intravenous fluids and who becomes short of breath or dyspneic should have the rate of fluid flow (increased, left the same, decreased).

decreased

182. When fluids are being given intravenously to infants and children, accurate intake is essential. The rate of adminis-

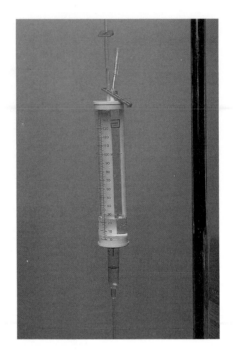

FIGURE **2-3**
Volume control
device. From Potter
PA, Perry AG:
*Fundamentals of
nursing,* ed 5, St
Louis, 2001, Mosby.

tration of the fluids must be kept constant. Therefore some type of volume control device is used with infants and children (Figure 2-3). Even a very small error in infusion could cause serious problems. Rates in children generally vary from 5 to 80 ml/hr depending on the size of the child, whereas the rate for an adolescent or adult could be 80 to 150 ml/hr. Fluid replacement for children depends on their age and body weight.

5   Rate for intravenous fluids in a child varies from ____ to 80 ml/hr.

Calculating the Rate of Flow

183. The rate of intravenous administration of fluids can be calculated when the drop size for the administration set being used is known. The size of the drops varies in the different parenteral administration sets. Generally they are 10, 15, or 20 (macro) or 60 (micro) gtt/ml. The nurse should know how many drops are needed to give 1 ml (1 cc) with the administration set being used. The variation in size of drops will differ among the various commercial administration sets. Nurses should always check the parenteral administration set box for the drop (gtt) size at the institution where they work. Microdrip tubing is generally used when small or precise volumes are to be infused.

Macrodrip tubing should be used when large quantities or faster rates are necessary.

The best action for the nurse to take when calculating an IV administration is to _____ for the drop rate.

184. The physician will prescribe an IV order for a patient. An example of a physician's order might be as follows: IV of .9% NaCl to run at 100 cc/hr. The first step is to decide whether you need to obtain a 250-cc, 500-cc, or 1000-cc IV bag of .9% NaCl solution. If you are to administer 100 cc in 1 hour, it is probably best to administer a 1000-cc or larger size bag of solution.

The next step is to determine the IV administration set to be used. Using the formula of drop factor (gtt/ml) divided by minutes (min) multiplied by volume (ml or cc), you would determine the drops per minute (gtt/min). Although microtubing would be appropriate to use in the example of administering .9% NaCl at 100 cc/hr, macrotubing might be a better choice because then you would be infusing 100 cc in an hour. Using a macrodrop tubing of 15 gtt/ml, you would calculate the drops per minute as follows: Divide 15 gtt/ml by 60 minutes (1 hour) and then multiply the answer by 100 cc (ml) (see Figure 2-5).

$$15 \text{ gtt/ml} \div 60 \text{ min} = \frac{1}{4} \text{ gtt/ml/min}$$
$$\frac{1}{4} \text{ gtt/ml/min} \times 100 \text{ ml} = 25 \text{ gtt/min}$$

a. If the administration set delivers 15 gtt/ml of fluid and the physician has ordered 120 cc/hr, the patient will be receiving ___ gtt/min.

30

b. If we use a drop factor of 60 and the amount to be infused is 50 ml/hr, the patient will receive ___ gtt/min.

50

c. If we use an administration set with a drop factor of 10 gtt/ml, and the physician has ordered 120 cc/hr, the gtt/min will be ___.

20

185. Now suppose the physician order reads infuse 1000 ml of fluid in 8 hours. Before being able to determine the gtt/min, we must first find out how many milliliters per hour are desired.

$$1000 \text{ ml} \div 8 \text{ hr} = \_\_\_ \text{ ml/hr}$$

125

186. Once you know the milliliters per hour (ml/hr) to be infused, you can use that number to calculate the drops per minute (gtt/min) to be given. If we found that 1000 ml divided by 8 hr is equal to 125 ml/hr, we could then determine the gtt/min

to be given by first choosing an administration set and finding out the drop factor identified on the box. For example, if we used an administration set with the drop factor of 15 gtt/ml, we would calculate that 15 gtt/ml divided by 60 min would equal ¼ gtt/ml/min and then multiply that by 125 ml, which would equal 31.2 gtt/min. Because we cannot deliver a fraction of a drop, we would set the IV rate at 31 gtt/min.

Using a drop factor of 15 gtt/ml, the number of drops per minute necessary to give 1000 ml of fluid in 8 hours is

31 gtt/min   _____.

187. We have an order to give 1200 ml of fluid in 24 hours. If the administration set requires 60 gtt/ml, how shall we calculate the drops per minute required to give 1200 ml in 24 hours? Let us review.

Step A requires we find out how many milliliters are to be infused in 1 hour. Step B uses the formula of drops per minute divided by 60 min and then multiplied by milliliters (or cc) per hour.

50   a. 1200 ml ÷ 24 hr = __ ml/hr

1 gtt/ml/min b. 60 gtt/ml ÷ 60 min = _____

50   c. 1 gtt/ml/min × 50 ml = __ gtt/min

188. Many times IV infusions are placed on an infusion controller or pump that has an alarm system that alerts the nurse in the event of a change in the IV flow rate or the ability to deliver the IV solution. Many agencies require that all pediatric solutions and all IV solutions with additives for adults be administered through an IV infusion pump. Because the infusion pumps sound an alarm when a change is detected in volume, rate, or pressure, any patient whose fluid balance is unstable should be given an IV solution through such a pump as well. Generally these infusion pumps deliver 60 gtt/ml. The nurse should check the agency's policy regarding IV infusion and receive in-service instruction on the use of the IV infusion controller or pump at the agency where he/she is employed.

the agency policy   To deliver the right medication to the right patient at
regarding infusion   the right dose and time by the right route, the nurse must
and/or controller   be aware of _____
pumps   _____.

Mechanical Factors Affecting Flow Rate

189. A change in needle position may alter the flow rate. If the bevel of the needle is against the wall of the vein, the rate will be slower than normal. A change in the height of the container of fluid above the needle site will alter the rate

as well. The greater the height of the container above the needle site, the faster the rate of flow.

   If we raise the container of fluid higher, the rate of flow will (increase, not change, decrease).

increase

190. If we keep the container of fluid at the same height above the floor and raise the level of the patient's bed, the flow rate will _____.

decrease

191. The patency of the needle will alter the flow rate. A change in the position of the limb may also affect the flow rate. It is best to avoid areas that are painful to palpation or are likely to interfere with a patient's activities of daily living when choosing an IV placement site. IVs inserted in the dominant hand or antecubital space are generally at risk.

   An IV inserted in the nondominant arm is at _____ risk for altering the flow rate.

greater

192. Mechanical factors that influence the flow rate of intravenous fluids include the following:

   a. _____

change in needle position

   b. _____

patency of needle

   c. _____

change in position of limb

   d. _____

change in height of bottle above patient

Adjusting Rate of Flow

193. Since the intravenous infusion is most effective when spaced over a long period, the infusion rate must remain nearly constant (except in emergency situations). However, after the rate is adjusted, continuous supervision is required to see that it does not change because of mechanical factors. In adults the rate should be checked at least every hour. In infants and children the rate should be counted and recorded every 15 minutes (Figure 2-4).

   a. In children the rate of intravenous infusion should be counted every __ minutes.

15

   b. In adults the rate of intravenous infusion should be counted every _____.

hour

194. If a liter of fluid is to be given over a period of 8 to 12 hours, the bottle or plastic bag should be labeled regarding how many milliliters per hour are to be administered (that is, 1000 ml 5% dextrose in saline to run for 8 hours). In

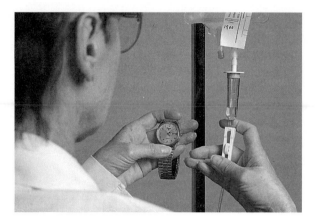

FIGURE **2-4**
Rate of infusion
should be checked by
watch. From Potter
PA, Perry AG:
*Fundamentals of
nursing,* ed 5, St
Louis, 2001, Mosby.

this way the nurse can tell quite accurately whether the rate is still adjusted correctly. A piece of tape or a label can be used to indicate the milliliters to be given per hour and where the level of fluid should be each hour (Figure 2-5).

a. If 1000 ml is started at 7 AM and is to be given over a period of 8 hours, _____ milliliters should be given by 11 AM.

500

b. By 1 PM, _____ should be given.

750 ml

195. Hypertonic and hypotonic solutions should be given at a slower rate than isotonic solutions. (Table 2-4 shows examples of isotonic, hypertonic, and hypotonic crystalloid solutions.) It is important that the nurse observe the patient for any signs and symptoms that indicate a reaction to fluid overload.

Patients who experience an increase in volume greater than they are capable of processing will feel short of breath. On auscultation the nurse can hear crackles in the lungs. Either one of these findings requires a severe reduction (if an immediate discontinuance is contraindicated as per physician order or pharmacy orders) or a discontinuation of the IV solution and the notification of the physician.

If fluid volume overload symptoms occur, the nurse should take the following actions:

slow the rate of
infusion

a. _____

notify the physician

b. _____

196. The maximum rate for administration of glucose to normal adults without producing glycosuria is approximately 0.5 g per kilogram of body weight per hour (0.5 g/kg/hr).

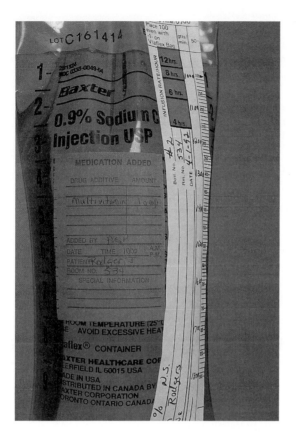

FIGURE **2-5**
Label IVs. From
Potter PA, Perry AG:
*Fundamentals of
nursing,* ed 5, St
Louis, 2001, Mosby.

At this rate it would take approximately 1½ hours to administer 1000 ml of 5% dextrose in water or saline solution to a patient weighing 70 kg (154 pounds), or twice as
long for 1000 ml of 10% dextrose. The exact rate at which
fluids are to be infused should be determined by the physician. A safe method of determining the rate of fluid administration is to divide the volume of fluid to be given by 24
hours.

    The safest method of fluid administration is to give the
fluids over a _____ period.   24-hour

197. If the rate of infusion exceeds the suggested maximum
rate, the body is unable to metabolize the glucose. Therefore it is excreted in the urine. This further increases the
output of fluid because more fluid is required in which to
dilute the glucose for excretion.

    The maximum rate at which the body can metabolize
glucose is ___ g per kilogram of body weight per hour.   0.5

✓ CONCEPT CHECK

The volume of urine output serves as a good indication of the adequacy of fluid intake in anyone with normally functioning kidneys. When there is a fluid volume deficit, fluids can be given orally or parenterally. The nurse is responsible for the administration of fluids and must be alert to the dangers when fluids are given parenterally. Dyspnea, increased respiratory rate, coughing, and cyanosis are symptoms that indicate an overload of the patient's circulatory system. Because the patient will benefit more from an intravenous infusion if it is spaced over a longer period, the nurse must know how to calculate and adjust the rate of flow.

✓ INFORMATION CHECK

1. At the morning report you are told that Mrs. Bottomley, a 53-year-old woman who has had a cerebral vascular accident, had a urine output of 400 ml for the past 24 hours.

24-hour intake
   Next you should find out her _____.

2. Mr. St. John, a 90-year-old man who was admitted yesterday, is receiving fluids intravenously. You note that his respiratory rate is increasing, and he is beginning to cough frequently.

check the 24-hour output
auscultate the lungs
slow the rate of infusion

   a. Your next actions are to _____, _____, and _____. Then notify the physician.

increased respiratory rate
cough

   b. Mr. St. John may have fluid volume excess, but you do not have sufficient data to determine additional, independent nursing interventions. The signs and symptoms you do have are _____ and ____.

3. Mrs. Emanuele, who is unable to swallow, is to receive 3000 ml of fluid intravenously. She will get the most benefit from the fluids if they are (spaced over a 24-hour period, administered very rapidly).

spaced over a 24-hour period

4. Caroline, who is 7 months old, was admitted to the hospital because of dehydration. The physician has ordered the intravenous infusion to be given at a rate of 50 ml/hr.

15 minutes
   You should check the rate of flow every _____.

FLUID VOLUME EXCESS

198. Just as it is possible to develop a fluid volume deficit, it is also possible to have an excess of ECF volume. Fluid volume excess is not likely to occur unless compensatory mechanisms designed to excrete excess fluid have failed.

Therefore fluid excess is not a disease state but a clinical manifestation of a health problem. The cause of fluid excess may be related to a diseased kidney, excessive secretion of ADH, decreased blood flow through the kidneys, or a decrease in cardiac output. Decreased blood flow through the kidneys and decreased cardiac output are associated with older persons. In the case of children, the cause of fluid excess is usually related to physiologic changes that fail to compensate for excess fluid.

Fluid volume excess results in a (wasting, retention) of fluid in the body.

retention

199. Just as in fluid volume deficit, the electrolytes are out of balance when there is a fluid volume excess. The osmotic pressure is reduced when there is an increase in the ECF volume because there is a decrease in the number of particles per unit of water. As a consequence, fluid moves from the extracellular compartment into the cell.

Therefore the cells (swell, shrink).

swell

200. Normally, when a person takes in an excess of water, water moves into the cells; this causes the osmoreceptors to respond, and the posterior pituitary decreases the secretion of ADH. As a result, the excess fluid is excreted by the kidneys. If ADH is unable to compensate adequately, water will be retained.

  a. Normally, excess fluid in the cells causes the posterior pituitary to secrete (more, less) ADH.

less

  b. When the secretion of ADH is decreased, the urinary output is (increased, decreased).

increased

Excessive secretion of ADH can occur as a result of fear, pain, or acute infections. It can also occur as a result of most anesthetics or analgesics, such as morphine or meperidine hydrochloride (Demerol). Any acute stress (such as trauma or a major operation) may stimulate excessive secretion of ADH. Postoperatively the excessive secretion of ADH may last 12 to 36 hours or longer. Accurate measurement of intake, output, and the patient's weight is important after any acute stress.

201. In a postoperative patient, fluid excess should be suspected if unusual behavior develops (that is, behavior different from that noted in the patient before surgery), if convulsive seizure activity or hemiplegia occurs, or if the patient becomes comatose. The water-excess syndrome that follows surgery or trauma is usually self-limited. However, if the person has any significant cerebral changes such as

convulsion or hemiplegia or becomes comatose, death may follow even though active treatment is given. The nurse must keep an accurate record of a patient's weight and fluid intake and output and must teach the patient to be alert for any changes and report such to the nurse.

Patients who are experiencing a new or acute onset of health problems are susceptible to fluid volume _____.

excess

202. a. Convulsions or hemiplegia caused by fluid volume excess are indicative of a (self-limited, serious) fluid volume excess.

serious

b. The effect of stress on the secretion of ADH is to (increase, decrease) secretion.

increase

c. This results in (increased, decreased) excretion of fluid.

decreased

203. An excessive secretion of ADH is likely to occur in which of the following patients?

a

_____ a. A patient who had a cholecystectomy 24 hours ago

b

_____ b. A patient who had a coronary occlusion yesterday and continues to have severe pain

c

_____ c. A patient who is receiving meperidine, 100 mg every 3 hours, for pain caused by a ureteral calculus

204. In addition to the situations identified previously, patients with cerebral lesions, lung cancer, or head trauma may have altered secretion of ADH. Monitoring a patient's intake and output is an important nursing function if the patient is suspected of having any health condition that alters the secretion of ADH.

As the secretion of ADH increases, the excretion of urine _____.

decreases

Impaired renal and cardiovascular function also are responsible for the retention of fluid volume. Whenever renal blood flow is low and the kidneys are unable to excrete urine, fluid volume excess is likely to occur. In persons with adrenal cortical insufficiency or acute renal insufficiency, excessive retention of water occurs because the kidneys do not excrete water.

205. In a patient with severe congestive heart failure or cirrhosis of the liver, conditions in which the body is unable to compensate for the increased blood volume and the renal

blood flow is low, the body's ability to excrete fluid is impaired. Therefore the kidneys are unable to excrete normal amounts of fluid. Water excess also can occur if large volumes of water are given rectally because the water comes in contact with the absorbing surface of the colon and is retained.

a. An excess of fluid volume is likely to occur in a person with severe congestive heart failure because of the decreased renal blood flow, which results in (increased, unchanged, decreased) urinary output.

decreased

b. Giving large amounts of water rectally may result in fluid volume (excess, deficit).

excess

SIGNS AND SYMPTOMS

206. Fluid volume excess can be prevented if the patient's total fluid intake and output are monitored. Changes in a patient's weight can be an indicator of the patient's fluid volume status. A 2% gain indicates a mild fluid volume excess, a 5% gain indicates a moderate fluid volume excess, and an 8% weight gain indicates a severe fluid volume excess.

a. If a person weighing 150 pounds gains 7.5 pounds this would indicate a _____ fluid volume excess.

mild

b. An acute gain in weight may be indicative of fluid volume (excess, deficit).

excess

207. As fluid moves into the cells, the cells swell. The symptoms that patients develop in response to fluid volume excess are the result of disturbed cerebral function. With severe fluid volume excess, the patient develops unusual behavior, has a loss of attention, appears confused, and exhibits aphasia. These symptoms may be followed by convulsions, coma, and death.

With fluid volume excess, symptoms resulting from disturbed cerebral function include the following:

a. _____

unusual behavior

b. _____

loss of attention

c. _____

confusion

d. _____

aphasia

208. A patient with fluid volume excess has warm, moist skin and may be flushed. The cardiovascular system remains normal as long as the excess fluid volume remains in the interstitial spaces or does not become too great. Edema may occur in dependent parts of the body or in

the lungs, especially if the person has congestive heart failure.

Which of the following may indicate fluid volume excess?

a
_____ a. Warm, moist skin
_____ b. Cool, dry skin

c
_____ c. Mental confusion
_____ d. Loss of weight

e
_____ e. Convulsions

209. A person with congestive heart failure who has a fluid volume excess will likely have symptoms that include edema of dependent body parts and the lungs. Edema, or fluid in the lungs, is the same symptom discussed in regard to fluid volume deficit occurring when fluid is given too rapidly and pulmonary edema results. The increase in volume increases the pulse and usually causes an increase in the blood pressure.

do
Patients with pulmonary edema (do, do not) have a decrease in respiratory effectiveness.

210. The hemoglobin and hematocrit, blood urea nitrogen

decreased
(BUN), and potassium levels are (increased, decreased) in a person with congestive heart failure because of the fluid volume excess and hemodilution.

TREATMENT

211. Fluid volume excess may be treated by limiting the patient's fluid and sodium intake and by treating the underlying health conditions and symptoms. How much fluid and sodium intake is restricted depends on the severity of the patient's health status. The physician will determine the amount of fluids the patient can be given. In infants and children, a proportionate amount of fluids should be withheld. The nurse should coordinate the administration of fluids with the interdisciplinary health team members from the dietary department and space the amount of fluid the patient can have over 24 hours. Any fluid restriction should be done in increments if possible.

In an adult with acute renal failure, the fluid intake

may
(may, may not) be limited.

212. Whereas fluid volume excess will likely be treated by limiting fluid intake, other treatment will be focused on finding the cause of the fluid volume excess. In addition to restricted fluid intake, sodium may be restricted and diuretics

may be used. Dialysis may be ordered in life-threatening situations such as renal failure or severe fluid overload.

If the fluid volume excess is serious, the fluid intake may be (restricted, stopped).

stopped

213. Any acute stress may stimulate an excessive secretion of ADH, which can lead to fluid volume (excess, deficit).

excess

214. This can be corrected before the excess becomes serious if the nurse collects the following data daily in susceptible persons:

a. _____

intake

b. _____

output

c. _____

weight

✓ CONCEPT CHECK

Normally, when excess fluid moves into cells, the secretion of ADH is decreased; therefore the urine output is increased. However, any failure of the compensatory mechanisms to reverse the fluid excess or any acute stress may stimulate an excessive secretion of ADH, which results in decreased excretion of fluid. With fluid volume excess, symptoms caused by disturbed cerebral function include confusion, loss of attention, unusual behavior, and aphasia. These symptoms may be followed by convulsions, coma, and death. The nurse must carefully observe patients likely to develop fluid volume excess and keep records of intake, output, and weight. In this way the excess fluid volume may be corrected before it becomes serious.

✓ INFORMATION CHECK

1. Mrs. Farrar weighed 141 pounds yesterday. Today her weight is 150 pounds. After determining that this is her actual weight today, the nurse should be aware that the gain may represent _____.

fluid volume excess

2. The nurse should look for symptoms resulting from fluid volume excess. Symptoms of disturbed cerebral function include the following:

a. _____

unusual behavior

b. _____

loss of attention

c. _____

confusion

d. _____

aphasia

3. A patient with fluid volume excess will have skin that is

_____.

warm and moist

weight gain

4. One sign or symptom Mrs. Farrar has that has been mentioned previously and supports the presence of excess fluid volume is _____.

restrict

5. The first step taken to treat fluid volume excess is to _____ fluid intake.

FLUID VOLUME SHIFTS

215. Fluids may shift from the intravascular compartments into the interstitial space. In some clinical disorders, depletion of the ECF develops because large quantities of fluid are held in an interstitial area, which makes them inaccessible to the body. This is called **third spacing,** and the fluid is usually essentially invisible.

not available

The term third spacing refers to fluids that are (available, not available) for use by the body.

216. This shift of fluid into third space may be localized to a single area or organ, or it can spread throughout the body. For example, a person with ascites will have large quantities of fluid in the abdomen. A person who has had abdominal surgery may have significant quantities of fluid that are not available for use by the body. The reasons why fluids may shift into third space include lowered plasma proteins, increased capillary permeability, or lymphatic blockage. These changes in the movement of fluids may be secondary to trauma, inflammation, or disease. The shift of fluids is a major factor in the fluid balance of people who have had abdominal surgery.

The factors that allow fluids to move from the intravascular compartment into third space include the following:

decreased
increased
lymphatic

a. (decreased, increased) plasma proteins
b. (decreased, increased) capillary permeability
c. _____ blockage

217. The first phase of third spacing is loss. Depending on the cause, it is likely to last 48 to 72 hours. During this time the symptoms will be those of a fluid volume deficit.

deficit

In the first phase of third spacing, you should expect symptoms of fluid volume (excess, deficit).

218. During this phase, fluids shift from the vascular to the interstitial spaces. The shift in fluids occurs because of increased capillary permeability in areas of inflammation and trauma. The increased capillary permeability allows

plasma proteins to leak into the interstitial space. In some situations lymphatic blockage may allow fluid to remain in the interstitial spaces. When fluids shift into third space even though intravenous fluids are being given, the fluid does not stay in the intravascular compartment, and the patient becomes **hypovolemic.** The person has a decreased blood volume.

When fluids shift into third space, the blood volume or intravascular fluid volume decreases. This is called _____.

hypovolemia

219. The clinical signs you should watch for with hypovolemia include decreased blood pressure and increased heart rate.
    a. In hypovolemia blood pressure will (increase, decrease).
    b. Heart rate will (increase, decrease).

decrease
increase

220. You should expect to find an increase in heart rate as the body attempts to compensate for the loss in volume by pumping the heart harder. The blood pressure will decrease when hypovolemia occurs. Hypovolemia also results in a low central venous pressure because of the lower circulating volume. The decreased urine output initially occurs as the body attempts to conserve renal perfusion.
    a. In hypovolemia the central venous pressure will be (high, normal, low).
    b. The urine output will (increase, decrease).

low
decrease

221. The second phase of third spacing is resorption. After the inflammation subsides, the fluid in the tissue spaces begins to be resorbed. Therefore intravascular volume will increase. Usually this shift occurs gradually, and fluid overload does not occur unless extra fluid is given at this time.

The second phase of third spacing is resorption; fluid moves into the _____ compartment.

intravascular

222. During the resorption phase, nursing observations and actions should be the same as those in fluid volume excess.

Intake and output (should, should not) be monitored closely during the resorption phase.

should

223. Hypovolemia also may occur because of a loss of blood, with or without the limiting of fluid replacement. As in the case of third spacing, the body attempts to compensate for the loss by conserving its perfusion to the major organs, and this results in a decrease in peripheral perfusion or a de-

crease in blood pressure. Subsequently, the heart rate increases in an attempt to add more blood to the systemic circulation and to support the function of the heart, lungs, kidneys, and brain. If left untreated, hypovolemia can lead to shock and result in the temporary or permanent loss of function of all the major organs, resulting in tissue hypoxia and eventually death.

can

Hypovolemia left untreated (can, cannot) cause death.

224. Treatment includes replacing fluids and establishing the underlying cause. The goal of the therapy is to help the patient regain adequate circulating blood volume, as evidenced by a normal blood pressure; this is done while supporting and preserving the oxygenation needs of the major organs.

to regain adequate blood volume

The goal of fluid replacement in hypovolemia is _____.

✓CONCEPT CHECK

After the body has been subjected to trauma, inflammation, or some diseases, fluid may shift from the intravascular compartment into the interstitial compartment and no longer be accessible to the body. This is called third spacing. The first phase of third spacing is loss, and it may last for 48 to 72 hours. During this time, the symptoms are the same as those for fluid volume deficit. The second phase of third spacing is resorption. Usually this shift of fluids back into the intravascular space is gradual. Nursing care is focused on observations and actions that will prevent severe fluid volume deficit during the first phase and on prevention of fluid volume excess during the resorption phase. The nurse must be sure to keep accurate records of intake, output, and weight. An accurate intake and output is especially important for infants and for elderly persons.

✓INFORMATION CHECK

1. When third spacing occurs, the shift of fluid during the first phase is (out of, into) the intravascular compartment.

out of

2. During the first 48 to 72 hours after trauma or inflammation, the patient's symptoms are the same as those of fluid volume _____.

deficit

3. The second phase of third spacing usually involves the movement of fluids into the _____ space.

intravascular

☙ KEY POINTS

1. Whenever loss of water from the body exceeds the intake, water is extracted from the extracellular compartment first.

2. When the volume of water is decreased, the concentration of sodium and other electrolytes in the plasma increases, which increases the osmotic pressure in the extracellular compartment.

3. In a person with normally functioning kidneys, the volume of urine output serves as a good indication of the adequacy of fluid intake.

4. Fluid intake should equal fluid output.

5. Fluid needs in children are based on their weight, age, or chronic or acute illnesses present.

6. Signs and symptoms of both fluid volume deficit and fluid volume excess can be assessed through the skin, mucous membranes, body temperature, lung sounds, heart rate, blood pressure, urinary output, neurologic changes, and weight.

7. The potential danger to the patient is increased when fluids are given intravenously because IV fluids go immediately into the systemic circulation.

8. Elderly clients and very young children may not have the ability to compensate and adjust to the changes in their fluid status.

9. Nursing actions are focused on careful assessment to detect changes in fluid volume before they become severe and to support compensatory mechanisms.

❓ CRITICAL THINKING QUESTIONS

1. Signs and symptoms of hypovolemia include:
   _____ a. thirst, hypotension, tachycardia, and decreased urine output.
   _____ b. bradycardia; full, bounding pulse; hypotension; and weight gain.

2. Signs and symptoms of fluid overload include:
   a. thirst, hypotension, edema, tachycardia, and cool, dry skin.

a

b

_____ b. shortness of breath, crackles, increased respiratory rate, and warm, moist skin.

3. Which of the following may be true about the effect of surgical trauma on fluid movement?
_____ a. In the first 12 to 48 hours after surgery, fluid in the interstitial spaces is depleted.

b

_____ b. Fluids may move from the intravascular space into "third space," causing hypovolemia.

c

_____ c. Areas of trauma and inflammation will have increased capillary permeability.

4. If you want to expand the intravascular compartment but contract the intracellular volume, what type of intravenous

slightly hypertonic

solution would be best? _____

5. Alexandra, a 4-month-old infant, has been admitted to the hospital with a history of vomiting and diarrhea for 5 days. She is dehydrated and has a rectal temperature of 104° F. Her skin is dry, and her respirations are rapid and shallow, with a rate of 68/min. Her apical heart rate is 164 beats/min. Her fontanel is depressed. An intravenous infusion has been started in a scalp vein. Alexandra's vomiting and frequent loose stools continue.

decreased

a. You would expect her weight to be (increased, decreased) from her pre-illness weight.

b. You would expect her serum sodium level to be (in-

increased

creased, decreased) from the normal.

c. If untreated, Alexandra could have a convulsion and have impaired respirations that would require that an endotracheal tube be inserted and that she be put on a ventilator.

severe

Her fluid volume deficit is (mild, severe).

d. Alexandra has a fluid volume deficit related to exces-

T 104° F

sive loss of fluid as evidenced by _____,

dry skin
respirations 68
fontanel depressed

_____, _____, _____, and

heart rate 164

_____.

6. Mr. Spinelli, age 82, has been admitted to the hospital for possible surgery to correct a urinary tract obstruction. He has been unable to void for the past 12 hours and has had urgency and frequency for several weeks.
a. If Mr. Spinelli has signs of fluid volume overload, his

may

heart rate (may, may not) be elevated.

increased

b. You would expect his weight to have (increased, decreased).

    c. If Mr. Spinelli has water intoxication and his extracel-
       lular fluid is hypotonic, you (would, would not) see
       changes in his mental status.

    d. The nurse will continue to assess Mr. Spinelli for changes
       in his signs and symptoms and will collaborate with his
       _____.

would

physician

7. Mrs. Niddrie, a 62-year-old woman, was hospitalized after a
   motor vehicle accident. Two days ago she had surgery to repair a perforated colon and duodenum. She has a nasogastric
   tube in place, and it is functioning well. This morning she
   complains of more abdominal discomfort. You notice that
   her abdomen is distended. When you take her vital signs, her
   heart rate has gone from 86 up to 116 beats/min and her
   blood pressure has dropped from 130/84 to 100/68.

    a. You should consider the possibility that Mrs. Niddrie
       may have a shift of fluid _____, also
       called _____.

    b. You would expect that her urine output has _____.

    c. Your nursing action will be to report the change to the
       physician. The signs and symptoms you will report in-
       clude abdominal distention and discomfort as well as her
       _____ and _____.

into the interstitial
space
third spacing
decreased

heart rate
blood pressure

8. Miss Jane, age 85, has a small bowel obstruction caused by
   adhesions from a previous surgery. Over the past 3 hours her
   nasogastric tube has drained 1200 ml of a brownish, fecal-
   smelling liquid. Miss Jane had been vomiting before coming
   to the hospital. For the past 3 hours, her urine output has to-
   taled 50 ml of concentrated urine. Her vital signs are pulse
   100, blood pressure 130/64, respirations 24, and temperature 99° F (37.2° C). She is confused and restless. She is getting an infusion of 0.9% sodium chloride at 100 ml/hr.

    a. These signs or symptoms indicate (hypovolemia, hyperv-
       olemia).

    b. Which of the signs or symptoms support your answer?
       _____

    c. What should you be prepared to do for Miss Jane while
       she waits to go to surgery?
       (1) _____
       (2) _____

       (3) _____

       (4) _____

hypovolemia

Low urine output and
diastolic B/P

Provide comfort
Expect additional
fluids to be ordered
Assess for fluid
overload
Measure intake and
output

PART

ACID-BASE BALANCE/IMBALANCE

KEY TERMS

acidity (acidosis)
alkalinity (alkalosis)
anion gap
blood gas analysis
buffer system(s)
defense mechanisms
metabolic acidosis
metabolic alkalosis
pH
renal system
respiratory acidosis
respiratory alkalosis
respiratory system
tetany

INTRODUCTION

Acid-base disturbances are usually the result of an imbalance of the homeostasis of the hydrogen ion concentration in an individual's body fluids. Generally, everyone experiences changes in the acid-base balance of their body fluids throughout their lifespan. The compensatory mechanisms of a healthy individual's body make on-going adjustments to accommodate the changes. When an individual's compensatory mechanisms cannot adjust enough, the imbalance becomes a health problem. Even a small imbalance can result in significant alterations in an individual's health status; severe changes may become life-threatening. Just as with fluid and electrolyte imbalances, infants, children, the elderly, and those whose health is already compromised are at greater risk for acid-base imbalance than are healthy adults. Consequently, it is important that members of the health care team quickly identify and intervene when an individual's acid-base balance is challenged.

It is important to note that some of the signs and symptoms related to an acid-base imbalance are insidious and can be mistakenly attributed to other health problems. It would be advantageous for the nurse to identify clients who are at risk early on and to be vigilant in watching for behavior that may indicate an acid-base imbalance. An acid-base disturbance is not a disease process but rather a symptom of an underlying health problem that has not been properly corrected process by the body's normal compensatory mechanism.

is not
225. An acid-base imbalance (is, is not) a disease process.

226. Clients who are particularly at risk for acid-base imbalance are:

infants
children
elderly
those whose health is
already
compromised

a. _____

b. _____

c. _____

d. _____

HYDROGEN ION CONCENTRATION

227. An increase in concentration of hydrogen (H^+) ions makes a solution more acidic; a decrease makes it more alkaline. The amount of ionized hydrogen in extracellular fluid (ECF) is extremely small. The symbol **pH** may be translated as the power of hydrogen; therefore the "p" is lowercased and the "H" (the symbol for hydrogen) is capitalized.

 The power of hydrogen is expressed as ___.

pH

228. Additionally, the pH value falls as the hydrogen ion concentration rises and rises as the hydrogen ion concentration falls. (**Acidity** increases with a decreasing pH and decreases with an increasing pH.) The hydrogen ion concentration in body fluids determines the degree of acidity or alkalinity. A pH less than 7.35 is considered acidic and a pH greater than 7.45 is considered alkaline. Therefore normal pH is between 7.35 and 7.45.

 a. Acid-base balance of body fluids is determined by the concentration of _____.

 b. Normal pH is between ___ and ___.

hydrogen ions

7.35, 7.45

229. A solution is acidic, neutral, or alkaline, depending on the number of hydrogen ions present. When the number of hydrogen ions increases to a certain point, the fluid becomes acidic. We report the hydrogen ion concentration in terms of pH. Acidity increases as the pH value decreases.

 A pH of 7.1 is more (acidic, alkaline) than a pH of 7.6.

acidic

230. **Alkalinity** increases as the pH value increases. When hydrogen ion concentration rises, the pH value falls. Conversely, when the hydrogen ion concentration falls, the pH value increases.

 A pH of 7.6 is more (acidic, alkaline) than a pH of 7.1.

alkaline

231. An acid is a substance that can provide hydrogen ions or is a hydrogen ion donor. Hydrogen ions carry a positive electrical charge and are therefore protons. Hydrogen ions are indicated by the symbol H^+.

 A substance that can give up or donate hydrogen ions is a(an) ___.

acid

232. A substance that accepts hydrogen ions is called a proton acceptor or a base.

accepts   A base is a substance that (accepts, donates) hydrogen ions.

233. An acid such as hydrochloric acid forms a solution containing a high concentration of hydrogen ions when placed in water. Therefore it is considered to be a strong acid. On the other hand, carbonic acid is considered to be a weak acid because in solution it provides a low concentration of hydrogen ions.

high   In solution a strong acid releases a (high, low) concentration of hydrogen ions.

234. A base is a hydrogen ion (proton) acceptor. In solution, a base, or alkaline compound, forms hydroxyl ions (OH^-).

accepts   A base (accepts, gives) protons.

235. An acid donates protons, whereas a base accepts protons. In solution, a base forms hydroxyl ions (OH^-), and an acid forms hydrogen ions (H^+).

a. An acid donates protons and in solution yields

H^+ (hydrogen ions)   _____.

b. A base accepts protons and therefore carries a

negative   (negative, positive) electrical charge.

236. A solution at a concentration of pH 7 is neutral because at that concentration there are equal numbers of both hydrogen ions (H^+) and hydroxyl ions (OH^-), which combine to form water (H_2O). The H^+ and OH^- are completely balanced. An acidic solution has a pH value below 7; an alkaline solution has a pH value above 7.0. The ECF of the body is normally maintained within the range of pH 7.35 to 7.45.

alkaline   a. ECF is slightly (acidic, alkaline).
equal (balanced)   b. At pH 7, the H^+ and the OH^- are _____.

237. Under normal conditions, the body maintains within the ECF compartment a constant ratio of 1 molecule of carbonic acid to 20 free bicarbonate ions (Figure 3-1).

alkalosis   At a pH of 7.5, the body is in a state of _____.

238. When the pH goes below 7.35, some degree of **acidosis** exists because there is an increase in the concentration of hydrogen ions. As the pH becomes more acidic, the central nervous system becomes depressed, and symptoms varying from disorientation to coma result.

Acidosis, an increase in hydrogen ion concentration,
depress   will (depress, stimulate) the central nervous system.

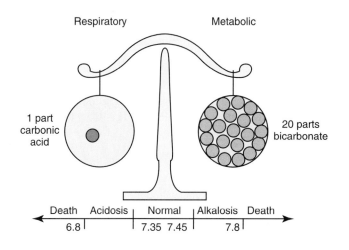

Respiratory   Metabolic

1 part
carbonic
acid

20 parts
bicarbonate

Death   Acidosis   Normal   Alkalosis   Death
6.8   7.35 7.45   7.8

FIGURE **3-1**
Carbonic acid–
bicarbonate ratio and
pH. From Potter PA,
Perry AG:
Fundamentals of
nursing, ed 5, St
Louis, 2001, Mosby.

239. When the pH goes above 7.45, some degree of **alkalosis**
is present because there is a decrease in the concentration
of hydrogen ions. Alkalosis causes an overstimulation of
the central nervous system. In alkalosis the nerve cells
may generate impulses even without the normal stimuli;
the symptoms may range from tingling sensations in the
fingers and toes to convulsions.

Alkalosis will (depress, stimulate) the central nervous   stimulate
system.

240. Slight changes in hydrogen ion concentration from the
narrow range of normal pH (7.35 to 7.45) cause marked
changes in the rate of chemical reactions in the cells. Some
chemical reactions are depressed, and others accelerated.
That is why regulation of the hydrogen ion concentration
is one of the most important functions of the body. The
more specific effects of changes in hydrogen ion concentration are discussed throughout the remainder of Part III.
a. The normal range of pH in the ECF is between
_____.   7.35 and 7.45
b. If the pH does not remain within these limits, the effect
on cells will be one of _____ or _____ chemical   increased
reactions.   decreased
c. Severe acidosis and severe alkalosis will result in
_____ if the imbalance is not corrected.   death

241. Thus far we have been considering the pH, or hydrogen
ion concentration, of ECF. Attempts have been made to
measure intracellular pH. However, it is impossible to directly measure intracellular pH clinically for the purpose
of treating an imbalance. The intracellular pH is generally

lower than the extracellular pH, although it varies in different organs. Intracellular pH varies in a parallel direction with changes in the extracellular pH. When an individual's blood gas is being evaluated, blood is drawn from the ECF. Therefore when the pH is measured clinically, this represents hydrogen ion concentration in the ECF.

extracellular   Clinically the (extracellular, intracellular) fluid is used in measuring pH.

✓ CONCEPT CHECK

The concentration of hydrogen ions determines the acidity or alkalinity of body fluids. The hydrogen ion concentration is indicated by pH. At pH 7.0, the hydrogen ions and hydroxyl ions are balanced, and the solution is neutral. The pH rises above 7.0 in an alkaline solution. An acidic solution has a pH below 7.0. The normal pH of body fluids is between pH 7.35 and 7.45. If the pH of body fluids goes beyond these limits, some chemical reactions in the body will be accelerated and others will be depressed. Either severe acidosis or severe alkalosis will result in death if not corrected.

🔖 INFORMATION CHECK

pH

1. The term used to indicate a measure of hydrogen ion concentration is ___.

neutral

2. A pH of 7.0 is _____.

acidic

3. A pH of 7.2 is more _____ than a pH of 7.5.

increased
decreased

4. Slight changes in the hydrogen ion concentration outside the range of normal will cause a(an) _____ or _____ rate of chemical reactions in some cells.

DEFENSE MECHANISMS

242. We know that the normal pH range in the body is 7.35 to 7.45. When the pH goes down, acidosis exists because there are more hydrogen ions available. In alkalosis the concentration of hydrogen ions is decreased. Normally the body maintains the pH between the narrow range of 7.35 and 7.45, even though it is constantly adding acids and bases derived from metabolism and from ingested food and fluids; this maintenance of pH creates homeostasis.

Acids
bases

_____ and _____ are constantly being added to maintain homeostasis.

243. To maintain acid-base balance, the body has three lines of defense that are compensatory mechanisms: the buffer system, the respiratory system, and the renal system.

_____, _____ and _____ _____ are the three mechanisms the body uses to maintain an acid-base balance.

Buffer system
respiratory system
renal system

244. The **buffer system** can respond within a fraction of a second to prevent excessive changes in the hydrogen ion concentration. The **respiratory system** can readjust the concentration in 1 to 3 minutes after a sudden change has occurred. Although the kidneys are the most powerful of the control mechanisms, if working alone, they would require from several hours to a day or more to readjust the hydrogen ion concentration after a sudden change. Each of the mechanisms shares the responsibility of maintaining normal hydrogen ion concentration.

The goal of the **defense mechanisms** is to maintain (normal, abnormal) hydrogen ion concentration.

normal

THE BUFFER SYSTEM

245. A buffer may be regarded as a chemical sponge. Depending on the circumstances, the sponge can soak up surplus hydrogen ions or release them. An acid-base buffer is a solution of two or more chemical compounds that prevents excessive changes in the hydrogen ion concentration when either an acid or a base is added to the solution. For example, if only a few drops of concentrated hydrochloric acid are added to a beaker of pure water (pH 7), the pH of the water may immediately fall as low as 1. However, if a satisfactory buffer is present, the hydrochloric acid will combine with the buffer and the pH will fall only slightly.
a. The pH falls when the hydrogen ion concentration (increases, decreases).

increases

b. An acid-base buffer should prevent excessive changes in _____.

pH (hydrogen ion
concentration)

246. There are four main buffer system(s) in the body that help to maintain the constancy of the pH. These major buffer systems are the bicarbonate-carbonic acid system, the phosphate system, the protein system, and the hemoglobin system. The bicarbonate-carbonic acid buffer system, although not very powerful, is as important as the combination of all the other buffer systems in the body. This

system is unique because each of the two elements of this system can be regulated: the carbon dioxide content regulated by the respiratory system and the bicarbonate ion content regulated by the kidneys.

The most important buffer in the body is the

bicarbonate–carbonic
acid

_____ system.

247. The primary buffer system, the bicarbonate-carbonic acid system, is also called the carbonate system. It consists of a mixture of carbonic acid (H_2CO_3) and sodium bicarbonate ($NaHCO_3$) in the same solution.

carbonic acid
sodium bicarbonate

The mixture of _____ and _____ makes up the bicarbonate-carbonic acid system.

248. Carbonic acid (H_2CO_3) is a very weak acid; its degree of dissociation (into hydrogen ions and bicarbonate ions) is less than that of other acids. Most of the carbonic acid in solution dissociates into carbon dioxide and water, the net result being a high concentration of dissolved carbon dioxide but only a weak concentration of acid.

weak

Carbonic acid is a (weak, strong) acid.

249. Hydrolysis of bicarbonate (HCO_3^-) in solution yields the hydroxyl ion and thus increases the alkalinity in the solution. Normally, to maintain acid-base balance (pH 7.35 to 7.45), the ratio of carbonic acid to base bicarbonate is 1:20 (see Figure 3-1).

$$H_2CO_3/HCO_3^- = \tfrac{1}{20} = pH\ 7.4$$

There are also small amounts of potassium bicarbonate, calcium bicarbonate, and magnesium bicarbonate in the body.

To maintain acid-base balance of body fluids, there

20

must be 1 part acid to __ parts base in the carbonate buffer system.

carbonate

250. The primary buffer system in the body is the _____ system.

251. Carbonic acid is a weak acid because most of it dissoci-

carbon dioxide
water

ates into _____ and ____.

252. An increased amount of available hydroxyl ions will in-

alkalinity

crease the (acidity, alkalinity) of a solution.

253. When hydrochloric acid (HCl), a strong acid, is added to a solution containing sodium bicarbonate, the following reaction takes place:

$$HCl + NaHCO_3 \rightarrow H_2CO_3 + NaCl$$

   Instead of the strong hydrochloric acid, we have the (strong, weak) carbonic acid. Because the strong acid combines with the sodium bicarbonate to form a weak acid and sodium chloride, the hydrochloric acid that was added to the buffer solution changes the pH only slightly.

weak

254. When a strong acid is added in the presence of a buffer system, the pH decreases (slightly, greatly).

slightly

255. If sodium hydroxide (NaOH), which is a strong base, is added to a buffer solution, the following reaction will occur:

$$NaOH + H_2CO_3 \rightarrow NaHCO_3 + H_2O$$

   This shows that the hydroxyl ion of the sodium hydroxide combines with the hydrogen ion from the carbonic acid to form water and sodium bicarbonate.
   Sodium bicarbonate is a (weak, strong) base.

weak

256. If a strong base is added to a buffer solution, the pH will _____ only slightly.

increase

THE RESPIRATORY SYSTEM

257. Carbon dioxide is being formed continuously in the body by the different intracellular metabolic processes. For example, the carbon in foods is oxidized to form carbon dioxide. The carbon dioxide diffuses out of the cells and into the interstitial fluids and then into the intravascular fluids. From there carbon dioxide is transported to the lungs, where it diffuses into the alveoli and is exhaled.

   _____ is continuously being formed by different intracellular metabolic processes.

Carbon dioxide

258. If the rate of metabolic carbon dioxide formation is increased, its concentration in the ECF also will be increased. If the rate of pulmonary ventilation (respirations) is increased, the rate of expiration of carbon dioxide also

will be increased—which will lower the amount of accumulated carbon dioxide in the ECF.

  a. If metabolism decreases, the carbon dioxide concentration in body fluids will (increase, decrease).

decrease

  b. If the respiratory rate is decreased, the amount of carbon dioxide in the ECF will (increase, decrease).

increase

259. The respiratory system acts in two ways as a feedback system for controlling hydrogen ion concentration. The first way is to respond to the hydrogen ion concentration. When the hydrogen ion concentration increases (acidosis) in the ECF, the respiratory system becomes more active (increased rate and depth of respirations) and more carbon dioxide is exhaled.

increase
    An (increase, decrease) in the hydrogen ion concentration will increase the respiratory rate.

260. Second, the changes in respiratory ventilation (respiratory rate) alter the hydrogen ion concentration in body fluids; therefore the carbon dioxide concentration in the ECF decreases. Because more carbon dioxide is removed, less is available to combine with water to form carbonic acid.

$$H_2O + CO_2 \rightleftharpoons H_2CO_3 \rightleftharpoons H^+ + HCO_3^-$$

carbon dioxide
    Less carbonic acid is formed when less _____ is available. Therefore the pH does not fall as it would if more carbonic acid were present in the ECF.

261. When the hydrogen ion concentration decreases, the respiratory system becomes (more, less) active, and the carbon dioxide concentration increases.

less

carbonic acid   262. If more carbon dioxide is available, more _____ will be formed.

263. The respiratory mechanism for regulation of hydrogen ion concentration has an efficiency of 50% to 75%. For example, if the pH suddenly drops from 7.4 to 7.0, the respiratory system will return the pH to about 7.2 to 7.3 within a minute. The reason for this level of efficiency is that as the hydrogen ion concentration approaches normal, the stimulus to the respiratory center is lost. It is then that the chemical buffering systems, which were discussed earlier, will help return the pH to a balance.

The respiratory system is capable of returning the pH (partially, completely) to normal.

partially

THE RENAL SYSTEM

Because the kidneys can excrete varying amounts of acid or base, they play a vital role in the control of pH. The **renal system** regulation of body pH is a complex device for excreting varying amounts of hydrogen ions from the body, depending on the number of hydrogen ions entering the blood.

264. The renal regulation involves a series of reactions that occur in the renal tubules. They include reactions for hydrogen ion secretion, sodium ion resorption, bicarbonate ion excretion into the urine, and ammonia secretion into the tubules.

     The renal system controls the pH by (excreting, holding) a varying amount of acid or base.

excreting

265. In normal metabolism the body produces an excess of acids. To maintain balance, the kidneys excrete more hydrogen ions in the urine and therefore the urine is usually acidic.

     When more hydrogen ions are excreted in the urine, the pH of urine becomes more (acidic, alkaline).

acidic

266. When the bicarbonate ion concentration in the ECF is greater than normal, more bicarbonate ions than are needed to combine with hydrogen ions enter the renal tubules. Although the kidneys are able to excrete either alkaline or acidic urine, the urine is usually acidic.
     a. When this happens, the excess _____ are excreted by the kidneys in the urine.

bicarbonate ions

     b. When more bicarbonate ions are excreted, the urine becomes more (acidic, alkaline).

alkaline

267. In addition to the renal system acting slower than the respiratory system, it differs from the respiratory mechanism in that it continues to act until the extracellular pH reaches exactly normal. It is important for the nurse to realize that an elderly person who has a decrease in nephrons in the kidney may require more time for the renal system to achieve balance. If it takes a younger adult 6 to 10 hours to achieve acid-base balance, it may take 18 to 48 hours for an elderly person or anyone who has decreased nephrons to gain a balance.
     a. The respiratory mechanism for maintaining acid base balance has an efficiency of 50% to 75%, but the renal

completely

system has the advantage of being able to neutralize (partially, completely) the excess acid or alkali that enters body fluids.

more

b. The renal system in an elderly person may require (more, the same, less) time to achieve acid-base balance than (as) that of a younger adult.

268. By returning some substances to body fluids and excreting others, the kidneys can compensate in several hours for even large deviations from the normal concentration of acid or base.

hydrogen ions

a. If the pH of ECF goes down, the kidneys will eliminate more (hydrogen ions, bicarbonate ions) to achieve balance.

bicarbonate ions

b. If the ECF pH goes up, the kidneys will eliminate more (hydrogen ions, bicarbonate ions) to attain balance.

✓**CONCEPT CHECK**

The homeostatic mechanisms are responsible for maintaining the electrolyte balance when a person is healthy. When a person's compensatory mechanisms are not adequate to create a balance, an alteration in health will occur. Subsequently an alteration in health may be related to the dysfunction of one of the regulating mechanisms or an increase in either an acid or base that is too great for the body to correct without treatment.

The body has three mechanisms for the regulation of acid-base balance: the buffer system, the respiratory system, and the renal system (Table 3-1). The buffer system involves two or more compounds that prevent excessive changes in the pH of body fluids. The most important buffer is the bicarbonate-carbonic acid system. Carbonic acid is weak and ionizes to a limited extent.

$$H_2CO_3 \rightleftharpoons H^+ + HCO_3^-$$

Bicarbonate is a weak base and yields the hydroxyl ion.

$$HCO_3^- + H_2O \rightleftharpoons H_2CO_3 + OH^-$$

The buffer system is important in minimizing the change in pH.

The respiratory system helps to maintain acid-base balance through the control of carbon dioxide. When the amount of carbon dioxide in the ECF increases, the respirations are increased in rate and depth to exhale more carbon dioxide. If the level of carbon dioxide is low, respirations are depressed. When more

| TABLE 3-1   **Acid-Base Regulatory Mechanisms** | |
Mechanisms	Action
CHEMICAL MECHANISMS	
Protein buffers	· Very rapid
Extracellular	· Provide immediate response to changing conditions
Albumin	· Can handle relatively small fluctuations in hydrogen
Globulins	ion production and elimination encountered under
Intracellular	normal metabolic and health conditions
Hemoglobin	
Chemical buffers	
Extracellular	
Bicarbonate	
Intracellular	
Phosphate	
Bicarbonate	
RESPIRATORY MECHANISMS	
Increased hydrogen ions	· Primarily assist buffering systems when the fluctuation
	of hydrogen ion concentration is acute
Increased carbon dioxide	· Stimulates central respiratory neurons, leading to increased rate and depth of breathing, causing more carbon dioxide to be lost and decreasing the hydrogen ion concentration
Decreased hydrogen ions	
Decreased carbon dioxide	· Inhibits central respiratory neurons, leading to decreased rate and depth of breathing, causing normally produced carbon dioxide to be retained, increasing the hydrogen ion concentration
RENAL MECHANISMS	
Mechanisms to decrease pH	· Most powerful regulator of acid-base balance
Increased renal excretion of	· Respond to large or chronic fluctuations in hydrogen
bicarbonate	ion production or elimination
Increased renal reabsorption of	
hydrogen ions	
Mechanisms to increase pH	
Decreased renal excretion of	
bicarbonate	
Decreased renal reabsorption	
of hydrogen ions	

From Ignatavicius D, Workman M, Mishler M: *Medical-surgical nursing across the health care continuum*, ed 3, Philadelphia, 1999, WB Saunders.

carbon dioxide is removed, less is available to combine with water to form carbonic acid.

The kidneys can eliminate either hydrogen ions or bicarbonate ions from body fluids and in this way can increase or decrease the pH. The renal mechanism requires more time to do this than the other systems, but it is more efficient.

INFORMATION CHECK

1. The defenses the body uses to maintain acid-base balance are as follows:

the buffer system   a. _____

the respiratory system   b. _____

the renal system   c. _____

2. The most important chemical buffer system in the body is

carbonate system   the _____.

3. When a strong acid is added in the presence of a buffer sys-

decreased slightly   tem, the pH is _____.

4. When the hydrogen ion concentration in the ECF increases,

more active   the respiratory system becomes _____.

excrete more   5. When the bicarbonate concentration in the ECF is greater

bicarbonate ions   than normal, the kidneys _____.

CLINICAL CONDITIONS OF IMBALANCE

269. Any factor that decreases the rate of pulmonary ventilation will increase the concentration of dissolved carbon dioxide, carbonic acid, and hydrogen ions.

acidosis   The result of this decrease is (acidosis, alkalosis).

RESPIRATORY ACIDOSIS

270. **Respiratory acidosis** is caused by any clinical situation, either chronic or acute, that interferes with ventilation, perfusion, or pulmonary gas exchange, thus causing retention of carbon dioxide, resulting in an increase in the blood carbonic acid and hence respiratory acidosis.

    a. In chronic obstructive pulmonary disease there is obstruction and less surface area to adequately exchange oxygen and carbon dioxide. This causes a retention of carbon dioxide, resulting in an increase of

carbonic acid   _____ in the ECF.

more   b. The pH of the ECF becomes (more, less) acid than normal.

271. The normal balance of carbonic acid and base bicarbonate is shown in Figure 3-1.

    Figure 3-2 shows an imbalance caused by disease involving the lungs.

    Because of disease, carbon dioxide is retained in the

carbonic acid   body; thus there is more _____ in the ECF.

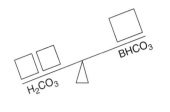

FIGURE **3-2**
Retention of carbon dioxide.

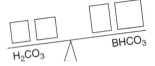

FIGURE **3-3**
Kidneys conserve base bicarbonate.

272. As the pH drops below normal range, the kidneys try to compensate by retaining more bicarbonate (base) in an attempt to raise the pH. Additionally, the kidneys excrete hydrogen ions (Figure 3-3). The urine then becomes _____.

    acidic

273. If the body's regulating compensatory mechanisms succeed in maintaining balance, the acidosis will be compensated or _____.

    corrected

274. Patients who have chronic lung diseases will have chronic respiratory acidosis. In chronic cases, the kidneys have time to compensate for the acidosis. However, with an acute respiratory insult, such as an airway obstruction and the resulting acute respiratory acidosis, the kidneys, which usually require hours or days to compensate for an imbalance, will have less of an opportunity to correct the imbalance. If the imbalance cannot be corrected by the regulating mechanisms of the body, then medical therapy will be necessary. _____ respiratory acidosis allows the kidneys time to compensate adequately.

    Chronic

275. Treating respiratory acidosis requires identifying the cause, that is, determining whether the problem is acute or chronic and correcting the acidity, if necessary, with medication containing a bicarbonate. This usually involves solutions of sodium bicarbonate or lactate-containing solutions given intravenously. If sodium lactate is used, the lactate will be oxidized to carbonic acid, allowing the sodium to react with carbonic acid to form sodium bicarbonate. Oxygen support and a mechanical respirator, if the patient's ventilatory function is poor, may be used to improve ventilation and perfusion.

base

If the respiratory acidosis must be treated, the patient will need more (acid, base).

276. In patients with respiratory acidosis, the problem or disease affects the respirations. Therefore the respiratory system is not available as a compensating or correcting factor. The buffer system and the kidneys can then help restore balance.

more

The kidneys compensate by excreting (more, fewer) hydrogen ions to return the pH to a normal level.

277. The problem caused by respiratory acidosis is excess carbonic acid that cannot be reduced by exhaling more carbon dioxide because the respiratory system is affected by a pathologic condition.

carbonic acid

Respiratory acidosis results from an excess of _____.

278. Any condition in which there is retention of carbon dioxide may cause respiratory acidosis. Signs we need to recognize in assessment that may indicate respiratory acidosis include distressed respirations, anxiety, disorientation, confusion, and body weakness. If the respiratory acidosis is severe, the person may become unconscious or may develop ventricular fibrillation.

distressed

a. One sign of respiratory acidosis is (easy, distressed) respirations.

disoriented

b. A person who has respiratory acidosis is likely to be (oriented, disoriented).

RESPIRATORY ALKALOSIS

279. **Respiratory alkalosis** results from a lack of carbonic acid caused by hyperventilation and a blowing off of CO_2. The decrease in $Paco_2$ will cause the pH to rise and alkalosis to occur. Respiratory alkalosis does not occur as often as respiratory acidosis.

carbon dioxide

Whenever there is excessive pulmonary ventilation of relatively normal lungs, there will be an increased loss of _____.

decrease

280. When excessive amounts of carbon dioxide are exhaled, there is a(n) (increase, decrease) of carbonic acid in the ECF.

281. Respiratory alkalosis occurs when pulmonary ventilation is increased, as in the case of anxiety or pain. Respiratory alkalosis can also occur in hypoxia (caused by high alti-

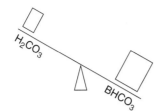

FIGURE **3-4**
Loss of carbon
dioxide.

tude, encephalitis, or fever) because of stimulation to the
respiratory center. Salicylate poisoning, such as from an
overdose of aspirin, and the use of nicotine and xanthines
such as aminophylline also cause direct stimulation of the
respiratory center.

    a. An _____ in pulmonary ventilation results in a respi-   increase
       ratory alkalosis.

    b. In respiratory alkalosis the body attempts to return the
       pH to normal levels through the buffer system and the
       kidneys by excreting bicarbonate ions and _____   retaining
       hydrogen ions.

282. Figure 3-4 shows an imbalance caused by hyperventilation.
      Respirations have increased, thus there is a loss of
      _____. The urine is _____.   carbon dioxide
                                                              alkaline

283. If the regulatory mechanism of the body cannot correct the
      imbalance, therapy will be directed at treating the underly-
      ing cause. Included will be treatment to correct the original
      condition, such as treating the cause of a high fever with an-
      tipyretics, treating anxiety with sedatives, or treating hy-
      perventilation by having the client breathe into a paper bag
      causing the patient to rebreathe the exhaled carbon dioxide.
      In compensating for the respiratory alkalosis, both the car-
      bonic acid and the base bicarbonate levels are decreased.
         The goal of the treatment for respiratory alkalosis is to
      _____ the amounts of carbon dioxide in the body.   increase

METABOLIC ACIDOSIS

Metabolic acidosis, a pH below 7.35, is a loss of bicarbonate
(HCO_3) from ECF or an accumulation of acids. Some causes
include severe diarrhea, vomiting, uremic acidosis, or diabetes
mellitus. For instance, in diabetes (Figure 3-5) the lack of insulin prevents the use of glucose for metabolism. The stored
fats are oxidized into acids. Acetoacetic acid is one of those
acids, and it is metabolized for energy. The acetoacetic acid
concentration in the ECF often rises to a very high level, and

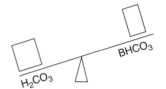

FIGURE **3-5**
Increased carbonic
acid.

large quantities are excreted in the urine. Metabolic acidosis occurs because of the high acid content in ECF and also because the acetoacetic acid carries large quantities of sodium as sodium bicarbonate with it into the urine.

284. Metabolic acidosis results because of the high acid content of the blood, or the loss of _____.

    sodium bicarbonate

    Patients with renal insufficiency or failure may suffer from metabolic acidosis because of their inability to excrete acids. In addition, medications such as potassium-sparing diuretics inhibit the excretion of acid.

285. Figure 3-6 shows the body's compensatory regulatory mechanisms attempting to correct the imbalance. Typically metabolic acidosis causes respiratory and cardiac symptoms while attempting to compensate as the lungs try to blow off CO_2.
    a. Breathing becomes _____

    hyperactive (deep and rapid)

        (Kussmaul breathing).

    carbon dioxide

    b. The lungs exhale more _____.
    c. The kidneys excrete hydrogen ions, and the urine becomes _____.

    acidic

286. In metabolic acidosis there is usually an ECF volume deficit that must be corrected by parenteral fluids. To treat diabetic acidosis, carbohydrates and insulin must be supplied. Intravenous solutions of sodium bicarbonate or lactate (such as sodium lactate) also may be needed to support the base bicarbonate, as well as fluid replacement and dialysis for patients with renal failure. Because of the changes in mental status, the neuromuscular system must be observed and the deep tendon reflex must be evaluated. Finally the patient's potassium level and ECG (electrocardiogram) must be monitored carefully. As mentioned earlier, serum potassium levels are elevated as hydrogen ions move into the cells and displace potassium.

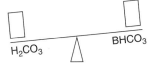

FIGURE **3-6**

Lungs exhale carbon dioxide. Kidneys excrete hydrogen ions.

Treatment is aimed at correcting the cause of the metabolic acidosis and replacing the _____ deficit.

base bicarbonate

287. a. In metabolic acidosis there is a deficit in available ____.

base

b. The homeostatic mechanisms that function to return the pH to a normal level include _____ _____.

the respiratory, renal, and buffer systems

c. The kidneys excrete _____.

hydrogen ions

d. Serum potassium levels _____ as the acidosis is corrected, and this may lead to hypokalemia.

decrease

e. In diabetic acidosis the respirations are called Kussmaul breathing. Because the respiratory system functions to return the pH to a more nearly normal level, the respirations become _____.

hyperactive (deep and rapid)

> **REMEMBER:** A patient with metabolic acidosis is considered to be a medical emergency. Because metabolic disorders are not as apparent as respiratory disorders, the nurse must be aware of any patients who are at risk and assess them frequently.

METABOLIC ALKALOSIS

Metabolic alkalosis may be caused by ingestion of large amounts of sodium bicarbonate or by the loss of acid through vomiting or gastric suction. Additionally, the loss of hydrogen ions, occurring with hypokalemia, as the kidneys attempt to conserve potassium, results in the excretion of acids. Diuretics, especially thiazide and loop diuretics, can lead to potassium, chloride, and hydrogen loss.

288. Normal balance of carbonic acid and base bicarbonate is shown in Figure 3-1.

a. Normal pH is _____.

7.35 to 7.45

b. In the carbonate buffer system, the ratio of acid to base is ____.

1:20

c. The symbol for carbonic acid is _____, the symbol for base bicarbonate is _____.

H_2CO_3

$BHCO_3$

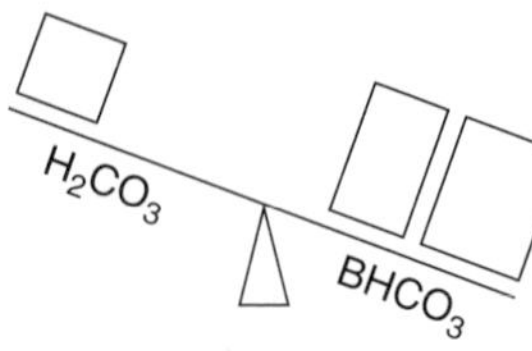

FIGURE **3-7**
Increased base
bicarbonate.

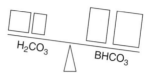

FIGURE **3-8**
Lungs retain carbon
dioxide.

increased

289. In Figure 3-7 base bicarbonate is (increased, decreased).

290. Figure 3-8 shows regulatory mechanisms.

slow, shallow
retain
hydrogen ions
alkaline

   a. Breathing becomes ____ and ____; the lungs ____
      carbon dioxide.
   b. The kidneys retain _____, causing the urine to
      become more ____.

291. If the body's regulatory mechanisms cannot bring about
balance, a chloride-containing solution can be given. The
chloride ions of the solution promote excretion of the bicarbonate ions and help to relieve the base bicarbonate
excess.

base bicarbonate

     The major factor causing an imbalance in metabolic
alkalosis is _____ excess.

292. Medical conditions such as Cushing's disease, which
cause retention of sodium and chloride and loss of potassium and hydrogen through the urinary system, may also
cause metabolic alkalosis.

conserving

     The lungs help to return the pH to normal by
_____.

COMBINATION OF TYPES OF IMBALANCE

293. We have considered respiratory acidosis and alkalosis and
metabolic acidosis and alkalosis as separate entities
(Table 3-2). However, it is possible to have a combination
of types of imbalance. For example, salicylates can cause
two types of acid-base disturbance. First, the salicylates
stimulate the respiratory center, which produces marked
hyperventilation and respiratory alkalosis. The salicylates
then cause a disturbance in metabolism, which results in

TABLE 3-2	Summary of Acid-Base Imbalances	
Type	**Cause**	**Compensation Mechanism**
Respiratory acidosis (carbonic acid excess)	Chronic lung disease Surgery Airway obstruction Pneumonia	Buffer system Renal system: excrete more H^+
Respiratory alkalosis (carbonic acid deficit)	Increased pulmonary ventilation Encephalitis Hypoxia Fever Salicylate poisoning Asthma Anxiety	Buffer system Renal system: excrete more HCO_3^-
Metabolic acidosis (base deficit)	Diabetic ketoacidosis Uremic acidosis Diarrhea Starvation Renal failure	Buffer system Respiratory system: rapid and deep breathing Renal system: excrete more H^+; retain more HCO_3^-
Metabolic alkalosis (base excess)	Excessive ingestion of base (antacids) Vomiting Gastric suction Excess aldosterone Steroids Diuretics	Buffer system Respiratory system: slow and shallow breathing Renal system: retain more H^+; excrete more HCO_3^-

increased accumulation of acids in the body and metabolic acidosis. When there is a combination of types of imbalance, treatment must be vigorous to prevent death.

It is possible to have a single type of acid-base imbalance or a _____ of types of imbalance.   combination

EFFECTS OF ACIDOSIS AND ALKALOSIS ON THE BODY

The major effect of acidosis is depression of the central nervous system. When the pH of the blood falls below 7.0, the nervous system becomes so depressed that a person is disoriented and later may become comatose.

294. The main effect of alkalosis on the body is overexcitability of the nervous system. This occurs both in the central nervous system and in the peripheral nerves, with the peripheral nerves usually being affected first. As a result of repeated stimulation by the nerves, the muscles go into a state of **tetany**, or tonic spasm. A patient with alkalosis

may die from tetany of the respiratory muscles. The symptoms of central nervous system stimulation are nervousness and convulsions.

depression
    a. Acidosis causes _____ of the central nervous system.

stimulation
    b. Alkalosis causes _____ of the central and the peripheral nervous systems.

✓ CONCEPT CHECK

Respiratory acidosis or alkalosis is the result of some disease or condition that affects the respiratory system. In respiratory acidosis there is interference, causing increased amounts of carbon dioxide to remain in the body. This results in an increase of carbonic acid. In respiratory acidosis the kidneys assume responsibility for correcting the imbalance by conserving base bicarbonate and excreting hydrogen ions.

In respiratory alkalosis there are decreased amounts of carbon dioxide in the body and consequently less carbonic acid. In this disturbance the kidneys excrete bicarbonate ions and retain hydrogen ions.

Metabolic acidosis is the result of a loss of base. In metabolic acidosis there are increased quantities of acid in relation to the available base in the intravascular fluid. Therefore the respiratory system compensates by initiating hyperactive breathing to exhale more carbon dioxide, and the kidneys excrete more hydrogen ions.

In metabolic alkalosis there is an increase of base in the intracellular fluid as a result of an excessive intake of base. Therefore both the respiratory system and the renal system contribute to return the pH to a normal body level. Respirations become suppressed to increase the carbon dioxide and consequently increase the carbonic acid as well. The kidneys retain hydrogen ions and excrete bicarbonate ions to return the pH of the ECF to a normal level.

TABLE 3-3 Summary of Normal Blood Gas Analysis

Blood Gas Components	Normal Value
pH	7.35 to 7.45
Po_2	80 to 110 mm Hg
Pco_2	35 to 46 mm Hg
HCO_3^-	22 to 26 mEq/L
BE	+2

pH, Power of hydrogen; *Po_2*, amount of oxygen dissolved in plasma; *Pco_2*, partial pressure of the carbon dioxide in plasma; *HCO_3^-*, amount of base available for neutralizing acid; *BE*, base excess.

INFORMATION CHECK

1. When carbon dioxide is retained in the intravascular fluid, the result is an increase of _____.

carbonic acid

2. An increase of carbonic acid in the intravascular fluid results in _____.

acidosis

3. When acidosis exists, the kidneys excrete _____.

hydrogen ions

4. In metabolic alkalosis more base bicarbonate is available; therefore the respiratory system becomes _____ and retains _____.

supressed
carbon dioxide

5. In metabolic alkalosis, the kidneys excrete _____ and retain _____.

bicarbonate ions
hydrogen ions

6. The major effect of acidosis on the nervous system is _____.

depression

NURSING CARE IN ACID-BASE IMBALANCE

BLOOD GAS ANALYSIS

295. With an acid or base imbalance, some of the effects are not very specific. Therefore the **blood gas analysis** is the most useful way to identify the imbalance.

     The most useful test for identifying an acid or base imbalance is the _____ analysis.

blood gas

296. Arterial blood is best for blood gas analysis. Arterial blood gas analysis (ABG) measures pH (hydrogen concentration), arterial oxygen (Po_2, the amount of oxygen dissolved in plasma), arterial carbon dioxide (Pco_2) (partial pressure of the carbon dioxide within the plasma), O_2 saturation (O_2 sat, the amount of oxygen bound to hemoglobin), and either plasma bicarbonate (HCO_3^-, amount of base available for the neutralization of acid) or carbon dioxide content. The normal range of arterial pH is 7.35 to 7.45; the normal range of arterial Po_2 is 80 to 110 mm Hg; the normal range of arterial Pco_2 is 35 to 46 mm Hg; and the normal range of HCO_3^- is 22 to 26 mEq/L (Table 3-3).
     a. The normal arterial pH is _____.
     b. The normal arterial Po_2 is _____.
     c. The normal arterial Pco_2 is _____.
     d. The normal HCO_3^- is _____.

7.35 to 7.45
80 to 110
35 to 46
22 to 26

REMEMBER: There are two very important facts about ABG interpretation. First, the P_{CO_2} is a measurement of the rate and depth of breathing, and second, when evaluating a patient's P_{O_2} and O_2 saturation, if either of these measurements are abnormal, interventions should be initiated immediately to improve the patient's oxygenation.

297. The arterial blood gases have the same normal values in children as in adults. However, infants have values that are slightly lower than those of children and adults. In a newborn (1 day old) the normal range of pH is 7.29 to 7.45, the normal range of arterial P_{O_2} is 60 to 80 mm Hg, the normal range of P_{CO_2} is 27 to 41 mm Hg, and HCO_3^- is 21 to 38 mEq/L. The P_{O_2} also decreases in elderly persons. A normal P_{O_2} in an 80-year-old adult is 66 to 74 mm Hg.

lower than
    a. In a newborn, the arterial blood gas values are (the same as, lower than, higher than) those in a child or an adult.

lower than
    b. In an elderly person, the normal P_{O_2} is (lower than, higher than, the same as) that of a child or younger adult.

    The measurement of base excess (BE) also is listed on an ABG result. The BE compares the bicarbonate level to a normal level. The BE is listed as either a positive or negative number. A low value indicates an acidosis, and a high value indicates an alkalosis. Normal range is +2.

298. When examining arterial blood gas values, you should look at the pH first. The pH is the prime indicator of acidosis or alkalosis.

acidosis
    a. A pH of 7.24 would indicate (acidosis, alkalosis).

alkalosis
    b. A pH of 7.56 would indicate (acidosis, alkalosis).

    You should look at the P_{CO_2} to determine the respiratory parameter. If the P_{CO_2} is increased, it indicates that more carbon dioxide is being retained. If the P_{CO_2} is decreased, it indicates that more carbon dioxide is being exhaled. A high P_{CO_2} indicates respiratory acidosis.

299. According to laboratory findings, the carbonic acid concentration cannot be measured directly in the hospital laboratory. However, the carbonic acid concentration is proportional to the partial pressure of the carbon dioxide, and this can be measured. The normal range of P_{CO_2} is 35 to 46 mm Hg. The average P_{CO_2} in arterial blood is 40 mm Hg, whereas the average P_{CO_2} in venous blood is 46 mm Hg.

In respiratory acidosis the P_{CO_2} will be (above, below) normal.

above

300. The next measure of the arterial blood gas analysis that will help you determine the type of acid-base imbalance is the base component. This is the metabolic parameter. The bicarbonate HCO_3 will be increased in metabolic alkalosis, meaning there is a greater amount of base than acid.
   a. The normal range for pH in ECF is _____.
   b. The normal range of P_{CO_2} is from _____ mm Hg.
   c. The normal range of HCO_3 is from _____ mm Hg.

7.35 to 7.45
35 to 46
22 to 26

REMEMBER: An acidotic state is signified by a pH lower than 7.35 and an alkaline state is signified by a pH higher than 7.45.

RESPIRATORY ORIGIN

301. After determining the type of imbalance, the next step is to determine the origin of the imbalance. If the origin is respiratory, then the patient's P_{CO_2} will be abnormal. Elevated P_{CO_2} means the patient is retaining carbon dioxide as a result of a decreased respiratory rate, which causes an increase in blood carbonic acid, hence respiratory acidosis. In the case of respiratory alkalosis, the P_{CO_2} is decreased as the patient blows off too much CO_2 by hyperventilating.
   a. In respiratory acidosis the pH is ____ and the P_{CO_2} is ____.
   b. In respiratory alkalosis the pH is ____ and the P_{CO_2} is ____.

low
high
high
low

The treatment for either of these two imbalances is to correct the respiratory problem. If the patient's respiratory rate is too shallow or low, oxygen therapy and treatment of the underlying cause is the major focus of the treatment regimen. Oxygen support will range from nasal cannula to mechanical ventilation, depending on the severity of the problem. Subsequently if the patient's respiratory rate is too high, asking the patient to rebreathe his or her own exhaled CO_2 will correct the problem. This can be done by having the patient rebreathe a mixture of his or her own carbon dioxide and oxygen from a large paper bag or by giving inhalations of 5% carbon dioxide at intervals.

302. The elevated P_{CO_2} must be reduced gradually. Mechanical ventilation is sometimes used to help reduce the P_{CO_2}.
   a. Mechanical ventilation may be used in treating respiratory acidosis to reduce the elevated _____.

P_{CO_2}

respiratory acidosis

b. Adequate ventilation is the main treatment for correcting a _____ imbalance.

303. The treatment of respiratory alkalosis is aimed at increasing the level of carbon dioxide.

CO_2

Treatment of respiratory alkalosis should increase the level of ____.

304. If oxygen is ordered when anoxia is present, it must be given cautiously to a person with chronic retention of carbon dioxide (such as occurs in emphysema). Oxygen may endanger the patient. Normally, as the level of carbon dioxide increases, the medulla and chemoreceptors stimulate respirations. In a person with a chronic elevation of carbon dioxide, the respiratory center becomes insensitive to the level of carbon dioxide. Respirations are stimulated instead by a decreased oxygen level.

increased

a. Normally respirations are stimulated by (increased, decreased) carbon dioxide.

oxygen

b. In a person with chronic retention of carbon dioxide, respirations are stimulated by low levels of _____.

305. At the beginning of Part III we learned that the respiratory system works along with the other compensatory mechanisms of the body to correct an acid-base imbalance. In the case of respiratory acidosis, as the respiratory rate increases to remove the large amount of CO_2 that is retained, the kidneys will conserve bicarbonate ions and excrete hydrogen ions to help achieve balance. In the case of respiratory alkalosis, the respiratory system is aided by the kidneys when they excrete more bicarbonate ions and conserve hydrogen ions.

increase
conserve
excrete

a. Respiratory acidosis compensatory activities are to _____ respiratory rate, _____ bicarbonate ions, and _____ hydrogen ions.

increase
excrete
conserve

b. Respiratory alkalosis compensatory activities are to _____ exhaled CO_2, _____ bicarbonate ions, and _____ hydrogen ions.

METABOLIC ORIGIN

306. An acid-base imbalance that is metabolic in origin will have an altered HCO_3 level. When the pH is lower than 7.35 and the bicarbonate level is abnormal, the patient has metabolic acidosis. When the pH is higher than 7.45 and the bicarbonate level is abnormal, the patient has metabolic alkalosis.

a. Metabolic acidosis is a pH _____ than normal with an abnormal HCO_3.

lower

b. Metabolic alkalosis is a pH _____ than normal with an abnormal HCO_3

higher

307. A patient with mild metabolic acidosis may have no symptoms. The acidosis is the result of a decrease in the alkali reserve. It may be caused by a loss of bicarbonate from the gastrointestinal tract or the kidneys or from excessive production of acid. The patient usually experiences general malaise or weakness, a dull headache, nausea, vomiting, and possibly abdominal pain. As the acidosis becomes severe, the patient will have changes in mental status.

Untreated metabolic acidosis will lead to changes in
_____.

mental status

308. Metabolic alkalosis is the result of excessive base bicarbonate and may occur because excessive base was taken orally or given parenterally. It also may occur when hydrochloric acid is lost from the body by vomiting or through suction. Therefore the symptoms we can expect because of central nervous system stimulation include paresthesias (abnormal sensations such as numbness and prickling), restlessness, confusion, and tetany.

The _____ of bicarbonate is responsible for metabolic alkalosis.

excess

Unlike the acid-base imbalances that are respiratory in origin, metabolic bicarbonate gains or losses are not visible but manifest themselves through other systems. These imbalances may be detected either by an abnormal arterial blood gas, by observing an alteration in a patient's central nervous system reactions, or by activation of the acid-base compensatory mechanism that is first to react—the respiratory system. Hence a change in respiratory rate may be the physiological manifestation for metabolic acidosis.

REMEMBER: In respiratory imbalances, the HCO_3^- is normal.

309. It is important to understand that although the patient may have an altered respiratory rate, it is not a respiratory imbalance if the ABG identifies a change in the HCO_3^- level.

The ABG blood result for a patient with a metabolic imbalance will show an _____ bicarbonate (HCO_3^-) level.

abnormal

310. A decreased pH stimulates the respiratory center to exhale more carbon dioxide and thus reduce the carbonic acid. Therefore, in metabolic acidosis, the patient will have respirations that are deep and rapid.

     Deep and rapid respirations that occur with metabolic acidosis (are, are not) a compensatory mechanism.

are

311. When compensation occurs, the pH rises slightly but may remain below normal. The P_{CO_2} falls because of hyperventilation. If the kidneys can conserve bicarbonate ions, the bicarbonate will rise toward normal (as will the carbon dioxide content).

     In partially compensated metabolic acidosis, the pH, bicarbonate, and carbon dioxide content return to more nearly normal but may remain slightly (below, above) normal.

below

REMEMBER: For balance, the body must have an equal milliequivalent (mEq) of cations and anions.

Not all of the anions are measured ordinarily, so the sum of the measured cations will be greater than the sum of the measured anions. The difference is called the **anion gap.** Evaluation of the anion gap may help determine the type of metabolic acidosis. The normal anion gap is approximately 10 to 14 mEq. The following formula may be used to determine whether an abnormal anion gap is present:

$$\text{Anion gap} = Na^+ - (HCO_3^- + Cl^-)$$

For example:

$$Na^+\ 140 - (HCO_3^-\ 24 + Cl^-\ 104)$$
$$140 - 128 = 12 \text{ (normal anion gap)}$$

312. When the anion gap is elevated, the acidosis is likely caused by organic acids such as lactate and ketoacids. The anion gap recognizes that there are anions in the body that (are, are not) ordinarily measured.

are not

313. Treatment is aimed at correcting the cause of the metabolic acidosis. In severe acidosis the physician will order fluids to be given to correct the base bicarbonate deficit. Alkalinizing solutions such as sodium bicarbonate or lactate-containing solutions may be given parenterally.

When sodium bicarbonate solutions are given, hypernatremia (excess sodium) and volume overload may be
complications of the treatment.

Treatment with parenteral fluids include solutions to
correct the deficit of _____.   base bicarbonate

314. Treatment is aimed at correcting the problem that produced the metabolic alkalosis by replacing lost acid in the
form of fluid or medication containing chloride. In metabolic alkalosis caused by vomiting, there will usually be a
deficiency of potassium also; so potassium chloride may
be ordered by the physician.

A chloride-containing solution or medication would
likely be used in treating _____.   metabolic alkalosis

General Nursing Responsibilities

315. We have considered the signs, laboratory results, and
treatment for the four types of acid-base imbalance. It
should be evident that overtreating one type of imbalance
may upset the balance in the opposite direction. We shall
now consider general nursing responsibilities in regard to
acid-base imbalance. The nurse must make pertinent assessments. These will include the patient's state of consciousness, degree of restlessness, type of respirations,
skin color, and vital signs. In observing the patient's state
of consciousness, the nurse will need to know whether the
patient is oriented, alert, or drowsy but rouses easily, or
whether he or she responds only to pain.

The nurse must assess the state of _____ of the   consciousness
patient.

316. In addition to the patient's state of consciousness, the
nurse should observe whether the patient is quiet or restless and the character of his or her respirations.

The nurse must assess whether the patient is restless
and what is characteristic of the patient's _____.   respirations

317. Thus far we have considered observation for state of consciousness, restlessness, and character of respirations.
The nurse should also observe the patient's skin for color
changes and check to see whether it is moist or dry.

In assessing the skin, the nurse looks for changes in
_____ and determines whether the skin is moist or dry.   color

318. The nurse should assess the state of consciousness, restlessness, type of respirations, skin color and moisture,

and vital signs. In taking the pulse rate, the nurse should look especially for irregularities in rhythm.

In taking the pulse, the nurse should be alert to

irregularities   _____ in rhythm.

319. In addition to making pertinent assessments, the nurse must protect the patient from injury. Because a person with acid-base imbalance may have either depression or stimulation of the central nervous system, the nurse must protect such a patient from injury during unconsciousness or convulsions. Protection of the patient from injury is an important nursing responsibility.

   a. In acidosis the patient will have depression of the cen-
unconsciousness   tral nervous system that could cause _____.

   b. In alkalosis the nervous system is stimulated, and the
convulsions   patient may have _____.

320. The nurse should make pertinent assessments, protect the patient from injury, and provide both physiologic and psychologic comfort.

The nurse should provide physiologic and psychologic

comfort   _____.

321. Another important nursing responsibility for patients with acid-base imbalance is accurate recording of intake and output. The type and volume of fluids taken, as well as lost, will be important in determining treatment. A record of intake and output is especially important in infants and elderly persons.

intake   An accurate record of both _____ and _____ is impor-
output   tant for the patient with either acid or base imbalance.

322. The nurse should make pertinent assessments, protect the patient from injury, provide comfort, and record intake and output. The nurse must also be able to perform the necessary therapeutic procedures as indicated. This might include catheterization and hourly analysis, venipuncture for diagnostic tests, administration of parenteral fluids, and other nursing procedures.

The nurse may need to perform therapeutic procedures,
hourly analysis   such as catheterization, for the purpose of _____.

✓CONCEPT CHECK

Acid-base imbalance caused by a disturbance in the level of carbonic acid is called respiratory acidosis or alkalosis. The laboratory criteria useful in determining the degree of imbalance are the pH and P_{CO_2}. In respiratory acidosis the pH will be low and the P_{CO_2} will be high. Treatment is aimed at relieving the cause of retention of carbon dioxide and then giving base or alkali to restore balance. In respiratory alkalosis the pH will be high and the P_{CO_2} will be low. Treatment is aimed at increasing the retention of carbon dioxide.

In metabolic acidosis and alkalosis, the problem is the level of base bicarbonate or alkali. In metabolic acidosis the level of base bicarbonate is less than normal, and therefore the acid side of the balance is high. The laboratory findings include a low pH and standard bicarbonate and carbon dioxide content. Treatment is aimed at correcting the cause of the imbalance and replacing base. In metabolic alkalosis there is an excess of base, which is indicated by a high pH and bicarbonate and carbon dioxide content. Treatment is directed toward supplying acid.

In both types of acidosis, respiratory and metabolic, the central nervous system is depressed. The nurse must be alert for symptoms such as disorientation, confusion, lethargy, and malaise. If the degree of acidosis increases in severity, the patient may become unconscious. In respiratory acidosis, respirations may be distressed. In metabolic acidosis there may be gastrointestinal symptoms of nausea, vomiting, and abdominal pain.

In both types of alkalosis, the central nervous system is stimulated. Therefore the nurse should be alert to signs of paresthesia, restlessness, confusion, and tetany. If the degree of alkalosis increases in severity, convulsions may occur.

The nurse must assess and report signs and symptoms that may indicate an acid or base imbalance. The patient must be protected from injury. The nurse also should provide comfort and keep a record of intake and output.

INFORMATION CHECK

1. Distressed respirations are likely to occur in and may produce _____.

respiratory alkalosis

2. A patient who has respiratory acidosis is likely to be (oriented, disoriented).

disoriented

3. In a patient with chronic retention of carbon dioxide, respirations will be stimulated by low levels of _____.

oxygen

4. In respiratory alkalosis, the P_{CO_2} will be ___.

low

metabolic acidosis

5. Nausea, vomiting, and abdominal pain sometimes occur in _____.

low

6. In uncompensated metabolic acidosis, the bicarbonate and carbon dioxide content are ____.

intake
output

7. The nurse should make pertinent observations, protect the patient from injury, provide comfort, perform therapeutic procedures, and record _____ and _____.

●● KEY POINTS

1. The concentration of hydrogen ions determines the acidity or alkalinity of body fluids.

2. The normal pH of body fluids is between 7.35 and 7.45.

3. The mechanisms the body has for regulating acid-base balance include the buffer, respiratory, and renal systems.

4. Buffers minimize the changes in pH.

5. The respiratory system helps maintain acid-base balance through the control of carbon dioxide and respiratory rate.

6. The kidneys can eliminate or conserve either hydrogen ions or bicarbonate ions.

7. Respiratory acidosis and alkalosis are characterized by an abnormality in the arterial P_{CO_2}

8. Metabolic acidosis and alkalosis are characterized by changes in the bicarbonate level or available base.

9. To identify an acid-base imbalance, evaluate the pH, P_{CO_2}, and HCO_3^-, and correlate them with the clinical situation.

10. The nurse must assess and report signs and symptoms of acid-base imbalance, protect patients from injury, and provide comfort to patients.

? CRITICAL THINKING QUESTIONS

1. You get a report with the following arterial blood gas results:

pH 7.16
P_{CO_2} 70 mm Hg
HCO_3^- 25 mEq/L

   a. The pH indicates (acidosis, normal acid-base balance,
     alkalosis).
   b. The P_{CO_2} is (low, normal, high).
   c. This P_{CO_2} indicates (acidosis, normal acid-base bal-
     ance, alkalosis).
   d. The HCO_3^- is (low, normal, high)
   e. The acid-base imbalance reflected is _____
     _____.

acidosis

high
acidosis

normal
respiratory acidosis

2. Another report with arterial blood gas results is shown
   below:

     pH 7.46
     P_{CO_2} 47 mm Hg
     HCO_3^- 34 mEq/L

   a. The pH indicates _____.
   b. The P_{CO_2} indicates _____.
   c. Does the P_{CO_2} correlate with the indication of the pH?

     ___.
   d. The HCO_3^- indicates _____.
   e. The acid-base disorder is called _____.
   f. With this HCO_3^- value, you would expect the pH to
     be higher. What prevented the pH from increasing
     more? _____

     _____

alkalosis
acidosis

no
alkalosis
metabolic alkalosis

Respiratory retention
of P_{CO_2} as a
compensatory
mechanism

3. Christopher is seen in the pediatrician's office with a history
   of vomiting. His blood gas report is as follows:

     pH 7.49
     P_{O_2} 88 mm Hg
     P_{CO_2} 35 mm Hg
     HCO_3^- 28 mEq/L

   a. Christopher's pH of 7.49 tells you he has (acidosis,
     alkalosis).
   b. His P_{O_2} of 88 is _____.
   c. His P_{CO_2} is (high, low, normal)
   d. The P_{O_2} is ____.
   e. The HCO_3^- is (high, low, normal)
   f. It is likely that Christopher has _____.
   g. Christopher's episodes of vomiting (did, did not) con-
     tribute to the metabolic alkalosis.

alkalosis
normal
normal
high
normal
metabolic alkalosis
did

4. Mrs. Stevens is seen in her physician's office with symptoms of polyuria (frequent urination), polydipsia (excessive
   thirst), tiredness, and muscular weakness. She is breathing
   deeply and rapidly. Her laboratory findings include glucose

and acetone in her urine and a blood sugar level of 560 mg/100 ml. Her plasma pH is 7.32, her P_{CO_2} is 35 mm Hg, and her HCO_3^- content is 20 mEq/L.

a. The client's pH of 7.32 indicates that she has (acidosis, alkalosis).

acidosis

b. Her P_{CO_2} of 35 is (low normal, normal, high normal).

low normal

c. Her HCO_3^- of 20 is (low, normal, high).

low

d. With her deep and rapid respirations, she will lose more _____.

carbon dioxide

e. Her rapid respirations are a defense mechanism to get rid of more CO_2 so there will be less (carbonic acid, bicarbonate).

carbonic acid

f. Since her respiratory system can assist in compensating for her acidosis, her pH is not as low as it would be without that mechanism. Her acidosis is (metabolic, respiratory).

metabolic

5. a. Which one of the acid-base imbalances would likely occur with a client with a history of chronic obstructive pulmonary disease (COPD)? _____.

acidosis

b. A client such as this usually has _____ than normal P_{CO_2}.

higher

c. Caution (does, does not) have to be taken when administering O_2 therapy to a client with COPD.

does

6. Jackie Angeli, a second year nursing student, has been studying for her medical-surgical final. She is a strong student but she is afraid she will not pass this test. As she gets ready to begin the test, her breathing becomes rapid and deep. Suddenly she says her lips and hands are numb. You notice that her hands are in carpal spasm. She says she feels as though she will faint.

a. You know that with deep and rapid breathing, more _____ is exhaled and lost from the body.

carbon dioxide

b. With less carbon dioxide available, there will be a deficit of _____.

carbonic acid

c. The acid-base imbalance Jackie has is _____.

respiratory alkalosis

d. The treatment for respiratory alkalosis is to increase the level of carbon dioxide. One way to do this would be to have Jackie rebreathe _____ _____ by holding a paper bag over her mouth and nose.

her carbon dioxide
and oxygen mixture

PART IV

ELECTROLYTE IMBALANCE

INTRODUCTION

Each electrolyte has special functions in the body. Although some electrolytes play larger roles than others, all are necessary for the function and maintenance of homeostasis and health. There are four basic physiologic processes for which electrolytes are essential: (1) promotion of neuromuscular impulses, (2) maintenance of body fluid osmolality, (3) regulation of acid-base balance, and (4) distribution of body fluids and electrolytes between the fluid compartments.

Here we shall consider the special functions of sodium, potassium, magnesium, calcium, and phosphorus.

KEY TERMS
hypercalcemia
hyperkalemia
hypermagnesemia
hypernatremia
hyperphosphatemia
hypocalcemia
hypokalemia
hypomagnesemia
hyponatremia
hypophosphatemia

323. The physiologic processes for which electrolytes are essential include the following:

    a. _____

    b. _____

    c. _____

    d. _____

neuromuscular function
body fluid osmolality
acid-base balance
distribution of body fluids and electrolytes

SODIUM IMBALANCE

324. Sodium is the major cation in the extracellular fluid (ECF). In fact, it represents about 90% of all the extracellular cations. Sodium ions are especially important in regulating the voltage of action potentials. Sodium is necessary for the transmission of impulses in nerve and muscle fibers. For example, if there is a deficit in the sodium concentration, there will be muscle weakness. Because sodium is the most osmotically active solute in the ECF, it is one of the main factors that determines ECF volume. Sodium and water go hand in hand, and, typically, where there is sodium, there is water. Sodium is primarily found outside the cell and is osmotically active. Therefore it plays a major role in controlling the size of the cell. When

sodium combines with bicarbonate and chloride, it regulates the body's acid-base balance. Normal serum sodium is 135 to 145 mEq/L

muscles
nerves
volume

a. Sodium is essential for the normal transmission of impulses in _____ and _____.

b. Sodium is also necessary to maintain the _____ of ECF.

fluid

c. Sodium, when combined with bicarbonate and chloride, helps regulate _____ balance.

325. Sodium is regulated by multiple factors. These factors include dietary intake, the pituitary gland hormone ADH, aldosterone secretion, and by the process of diffusion in the sodium-potassium pump. A person's sodium level depends on how much sodium is ingested daily. The average adult requires 2 g/day. Sodium is absorbed by the gastrointestinal (GI) tract and excreted through the kidneys and skin.

Dietary intake
ADH, aldosterone
sodium-potassium
pump

_____, _____, _____, and _____
regulate sodium balance.

326. The first regulatory mechanism we will look at is the sensation of thirst. When an individual's fluid volume is decreased, the sensation of thirst is activated to encourage an individual to ingest fluids. Thirst can also be initiated when an individual's serum sodium level is increased in an attempt to dilute the sodium/water ratio. It is important to note that any individual who is too young or who is cognitively impaired will not be able to express the sensation of thirst. Therefore it becomes part of nursing care to provide a variety of fluids at frequent intervals, provided there are no fluid volume overload concerns.

increase
dilute

Thirst is initiated to either _____ fluid volume or _____ serum sodium.

327. It is important to understand the antidiuretic hormone (ADH) in relation to sodium. ADH is either stimulated or suppressed according to an individual's fluid volume status. When there is an increase in fluid volume, the release of ADH is stimulated. If ADH is increased when there is already an increased fluid volume, the effect is simply to increase the fluid volume even more. So when the fluid volume is elevated, the stimulation of ADH is suppressed. If the body is no longer "holding," urinary output will be increased and hence the circulating blood volume will be

reduced. Opposite to this effect is the condition of fluid volume deficit, in which ADH is stimulated. In this case, ADH acts as a HOLD on excretion, thereby water is retained and added to the circulating blood volume. Once the serum osmolality is increased and there is sufficient volume, ADH is no longer needed and therefore is no longer stimulated.

ADH is either stimulated or suppressed according to the body's _____ status.   fluid volume deficit

---

REMEMBER: ADH places a HOLD on output. Let the *H* in ADH remind you of the word "hold."

---

328. The kidneys are extremely important in regulating sodium balance, primarily through the action of aldosterone. Aldosterone produced by the adrenal cortex stimulates the renal tubules to conserve water and sodium when the body's serum sodium level is low. Alternatively, high serum sodium levels inhibit aldosterone production.

     The hormone produced by the adrenal glands that is influential in regulating sodium balance is _____.   aldosterone

329. Normally almost all the sodium that is filtered by the kidneys is resorbed. Most of the sodium is resorbed with chloride, but some is resorbed when sodium ions are exchanged for potassium and hydrogen ions. In the absence of aldosterone, a person can become seriously depleted of sodium and chloride.

     Aldosterone is an important hormone for the regulation of _____ and chloride.   sodium

330. There are several factors that affect the rate of secretion of aldosterone. Any one or a combination of these factors stimulates the secretion of aldosterone and, consequently, the level of sodium. These factors include reduced blood volume or cardiac output, decreased extracellular sodium, increased extracellular potassium, and physical stress. Renin, which is secreted by the kidneys and causes the formation of angiotensin, also may act directly on the adrenal cortex to secrete more aldosterone when the sodium concentration is low.
    a. Reduced blood volume and cardiac output stimulate the production of _____.   aldosterone
    b. Aldosterone is secreted in greater amounts when the level of extracellular sodium is (high, low).   low

c. The secretion of aldosterone is stimulated by a (high, low) level of extracellular potassium.

331. In the elderly, renal blood flow decreases, cardiac output decreases, plasma renin activity is lower, and the stress response to sodium restriction is blunted. All of these changes that occur with aging affect the rate of secretion of aldosterone. This explains the increased vulnerability of the elderly person to a sodium imbalance.

more
The elderly are (more, less) likely to have a sodium imbalance than are children or younger adults.

332. The regulation of sodium in the body is very closely related to the regulation of fluid volume because the fluid volume can be adjusted by regulating the level of sodium in the body.

increase
Because of osmolality, as the sodium content increases, the volume of fluid will (increase, decrease).

The last regulatory system is the sodium-potassium pump. Using energy known as active transport, the sodium-potassium pump helps maintain normal serum sodium levels by moving sodium out of the cell into the extracellular space and keeping potassium inside the cell or the intracellular space. This balance maintains homeostasis of fluid volume and the electrolytes sodium and potassium.

SODIUM DEFICIT (HYPONATREMIA)

333. Vomiting, diarrhea, or GI drainage from suction or fistulas may cause a sodium deficit, less than 135 mEq/L, called **hyponatremia.** "Natrium" is the Latin word for sodium, and the symbol is Na. Although normally sodium and chloride are resorbed by the kidneys, sodium may be lost from the body through GI secretions.

a loss
Loss of secretions from the GI tract may cause (a loss, an increase) of sodium.

Causes

334. Sodium may be lost through the skin as a result of excessive sweating, burns, or cystic fibrosis.

skin
With sweating, as well as with burns and cystic fibrosis, sodium is lost through the ＿＿.

335. Although sodium may be lost from the GI tract or the skin, it may also be lost via kidneys. When medications that cause diuresis are given, sodium will be lost in the

urine. Another cause of hyponatremia is renal disease, especially salt-losing nephritis.

If the kidneys are unable to resorb _____, hyponatremia will result.

sodium

336. Hyponatremia also may occur when sodium is isolated within the body and is not physiologically available, such as when there is an obstruction of the small bowel and large amounts of fluid containing sodium are held in the intestinal lumen. It may occur in burns when edema accumulates at the burn site or in peritonitis when ECF is held in the abdomen. The sodium in such fluids is not available to the body for necessary functions.

Fluid containing sodium may be isolated in the body when any of the following occurs:

a. _____
b. _____
c. _____

small bowel
obstruction
burns
peritonitis

337. Hyponatremia may occur when there is a gain in body water as a result of excessive fluid intake, which leads to sodium dilution. Other causes of hyponatremia include heart failure, nephrotic syndrome, and cirrhosis of the liver. Drugs that may impair water excretion include nicotine, chlorpropamide (Diabinese), morphine, barbiturates, and isoproterenol (Isuprel). The syndrome of inappropriate secretion of antidiuretic hormone (SIADH) (which is the secretion of ADH even when the fluid volume status does not warrant it) may cause hyponatremia and severe water intoxication.

Whereas some diseases and medications may cause hyponatremia, fluid intake that is (minimal, normal, excessive) also may lead to hyponatremia.

excessive

338. Although both fluid and electrolytes are lost in the previously mentioned conditions that cause sodium deficit, the fluid may be more readily replaced, leaving only a deficit of sodium. For example, anyone who is perspiring heavily and drinking large quantities of water is restoring only the lost fluid volume, not the sodium, unless that person also replaces the lost salt (sodium chloride) as well.

Whenever sodium is lost from the body, the fluid volume will be (increased, decreased).

decreased

Signs and Symptoms

339. The nurse will assess for signs and symptoms that vary depending on the degree of depletion of sodium and water, as

well as on the rapidity of the loss. If the loss is severe and occurs suddenly, the clinical picture will be one of shock. If the loss is more gradual, the symptoms will include weakness, lethargy, and mental depression (Figure 4-1).

Weakness, lethargy, and mental depression are symptoms of sodium (deficit, excess).

deficit

340. Muscle weakness, fatigue, headache, hypotension, and vertigo may occur with a sodium deficit. Apprehension, confusion, and ataxia, as well as convulsions and coma, may occur because of increased intracellular fluid content. Muscle cramps may occur, especially if the fluid is replaced without the sodium, because fluid replacement intensifies the sodium loss. In the elderly these symptoms are often attributed to aging, and the hyponatremia may be missed.

Headache, vertigo, hypotension, muscle weakness, and muscle _____ may occur in those with a sodium deficit.

cramps

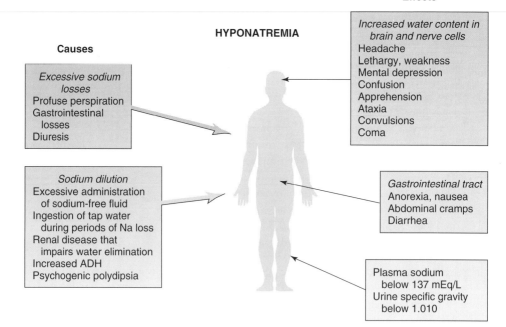

FIGURE **4-1**
Causes and effects of hyponatremia. From Beare PG, Myers JL: *Adult health nursing*, ed 3, St Louis, 1998, Mosby.

341. A person with hyponatremia also may have GI symptoms, including anorexia, nausea, and vomiting.

    A person with hyponatremia may have the following GI symptoms:

    a. _____   anorexia
    b. _____   nausea
    c. _____   vomiting

342. Because the level of sodium in the body also controls the ECF volume, some of the signs and symptoms of sodium deficit will parallel those of fluid volume deficit. There will be a loss of skin turgor; that is, if the skin of the arm is picked up and released, it will tend to remain stretched and folded for a half minute or more. Normally, when the skin is picked up, it returns almost immediately to its previous shape (Figure 4-2). In the elderly, skin turgor is not a useful sign of sodium deficit because skin loses elasticity with advancing age. However, in infants and small children loss of skin elasticity is considered a classic sign of dehydration.

    With sodium deficit, the skin will show loss of _____   turgor
    in children and younger adults.

> **REMEMBER:** Infants are more vulnerable to alterations in fluid and electrolyte balance because they have a greater fluid intake and output relative to their size (Wong, 1999).

343. The eyeballs may be sunken and feel soft on palpation. The tongue may be wrinkled and shrunken.

    In addition to a loss of skin turgor with hyponatremia, there may be changes in the eyeballs and _____.   tongue

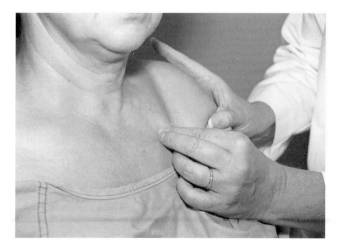

FIGURE **4-2**
Measurement of skin turgor. From Perry AG, Potter PA: *Clinical nursing skills and techniques*, ed 4, St Louis, 1998, Mosby.

344. The cardiovascular signs will vary with the rate and degree of sodium loss. There may be orthostatic hypotension, which is a drop in blood pressure when the person stands and which may cause fainting.

hypotension   Hyponatremia may cause orthostatic _____.

345. There also may be tachycardia, thready peripheral pulse or loss of peripheral pulse, and collapsed neck veins.

collapse   In hyponatremia the pulse may be rapid and thready and the neck veins may _____.

346. If the hyponatremia develops slowly or is less severe, the symptoms will be less dramatic. Be alert to the possible need for sodium in a person who is fatigued, has a loss of energy, and feels faint on arising.

Hyponatremia that is not severe may cause the following symptoms:

fatigue   a. _____
loss of energy   b. _____
fainting   c. _____

Laboratory Findings

347. The hematocrit of a person with hyponatremia will be elevated because of hemoconcentration, (that is, the percentage of red blood cells [RBCs] to fluid appears to be proportional even though in actuality the number of RBCs may be low), and the serum sodium will be low. Knowing the level of sodium is useful in differentiating sodium loss from water loss. In water loss a high hematocrit level is associated with a high sodium concentration.

above   a. In hyponatremia the hematocrit will be (above, below) normal.

below   b. The serum sodium will be (above, below) normal.

REMEMBER: In hyponatremia the serum sodium will be less than 135 mEq/L. The level of sodium does not change with increasing age.

348. The serum level of chloride or bicarbonate also will be low. The serum potassium may be high because some loss of sodium will cause increased retention of potassium.

low   The serum level of chloride will likely be (high, low).

349. In sodium deficit the urinary volume will likely be low, as will the sodium and chloride concentration in the urine. The specific gravity of urine will be below 1.010.

The urinary volume and concentration of sodium and
chloride will be (high, low).   low

Treatment

The aim of treatment is to restore balance by replacing the
deficit of sodium and water. For mild hyponatremia, fluid replacement and oral sodium supplements may be ordered. If
shock exists, parenteral sodium (3% or 5% hypertonic saline
solution) and water will be needed. Medications such as nor-
epinephrine (Levophed) or metaraminol (Aramine) will not be
effective until some of the sodium has been replaced.

350. The amount of sodium to be replaced is calculated by the
     physician on the basis of the serum sodium level and the
     weight of the patient. The rate of flow for parenteral re-
     placement must be carefully controlled because too rapid
     replacement will increase the loss of electrolytes. Unless
     there is circulatory insufficiency, sodium deficits are re-
     placed over a 12- to 24-hour period.
     a. If the hyponatremia is severe, replacement of sodium
        and water will be needed by the _____   parenteral
        _____ route.   (intravenous)
     b. The rate of flow for sodium chloride solution adminis-
        tered intravenously should be (rapid, controlled).   controlled

351. Another aspect of treatment is to stop further loss of so-
     dium. For example, if the patient is losing fluid from a
     pancreatic fistula, this fluid will have a high sodium con-
     tent. Therefore isotonic saline solution should be used
     to replace the loss. Additional sodium chloride may be
     necessary.
         Pancreatic drainage has a high _____ content.   sodium

✓CONCEPT CHECK

Sodium is the main extracellular cation. Some functions of sodium are transmission of impulses in nerve and muscle fibers,
control of cell size, and maintenance of ECF volume.

   Normal kidneys can selectively regulate the level of sodium
in the body. Reduced blood volume, decreased cardiac output,
low extracellular sodium, high extracellular potassium, and
physical stress stimulate the secretion of aldosterone, which
causes an increased resorption of sodium by the kidneys.

   All secretions from the GI tract contain sodium, which is
normally resorbed. Therefore any abnormal loss of GI secretions can cause a sodium deficit (hyponatremia). Sodium may
also be lost through the skin or kidneys. Sudden loss of sodium

may produce shock. Gradual sodium loss may be evidenced by symptoms of fatigue, loss of energy, and fainting. Other signs of hyponatremia include tachycardia and hypotension. The hematocrit will be above normal, and serum sodium will be low. Treatment is aimed at restoring balance by replacing the water deficit and the sodium deficit, often in the form of sodium chloride.

INFORMATION CHECK

sodium   1. The most osmotically active extracellular cation is _____.

all   2. Normally almost (all, none) of the sodium filtered by the kidney is resorbed.

increased   3. Reduced cardiac output will stimulate (increased, decreased) secretion of aldosterone.

potassium
hydrogen   4. When sodium is resorbed because of the effect of aldosterone, more _____ and _____ ions are excreted.

sodium   5. In peritonitis, in which large amounts of ECF are held in the peritoneal cavity, there may be a _____ deficit because this fluid is not available to the body.

increase the problem   6. In the treatment of a sodium deficit by the intravenous administration of sodium chloride, very rapid replacement may (be indicated, increase the problem).

low   7. In an adult patient who has been vomiting for 2 days, you would expect her serum sodium to be (high, normal, low).

8. Which of the following signs or symptoms would you expect to find in a patient who had been vomiting for several days?

a   _____ a. Fatigue
_____ b. Hypertension
c   _____ c. Weakness
d   _____ d. Loss of skin turgor
_____ e. Edema

SODIUM EXCESS (HYPERNATREMIA)

The kidneys regulate sodium excretion in a healthy person according to intake. If the kidneys fail because of hormonal or hemodynamic effects, excess sodium, greater than 145 mEq/L, (**hypernatremia**) may develop. When this occurs, there is also fluid retention, or edema, and therefore an increase in ECF volume as well. For the kidneys to perform their regulatory function, an adequate blood flow must be present as well as a normal aldosterone system. Therefore conditions in which hypernatremia may be a problem include renal failure (with sodium retention), inadequate blood circulation to the kidneys (as in congestive heart failure), cirrhosis of the liver, overproduction of aldosterone by the adrenal cortex, use of large doses of adrenal corticoids, greater than needed ingestion of food or drinks high in sodium content, or the lack of ability to respond to the sensation of thirst.

352. The kidneys must have adequate _____ and _____   blood flow
     _____ to regulate the sodium level.   normal aldosterone

Causes

353. We can say, then, that hypernatremia causes increased water retention and therefore an increased ECF volume. If a person has increased resorption of sodium but is unable to take in additional fluid, the concentration of extracellular sodium will increase. Usually, however, the concentration of extracellular sodium does not increase even with increased resorption of sodium, because the person drinks more fluid and therefore dilutes the retained sodium.

  If a person has an increased resorption of sodium and is unable to take in additional fluid, the concentration of sodium will _____.   increase

Signs and Symptoms

354. Symptoms of hypernatremia are caused by the hypertonicity of the ECF and the lack of water. Therefore the symptoms will be those of dehydration. The mucous membranes will be dry, the skin flushed, the temperature elevated, and the urine output decreased (Figure 4-3).

  If there is increased resorption of sodium without an increase in fluid intake, the symptoms will be those of

  _____.   dehydration

REMEMBER: Hypernatremia is especially dangerous in the very old and the very young. Signs and symptoms such as thirst and altered skin turgor may be more difficult to detect.

355. Normal serum sodium in older children and adults is 135 to 148 mEq/L.

  Normal serum sodium in children and adults is ___ to   135
  ___ mEq/L.   148

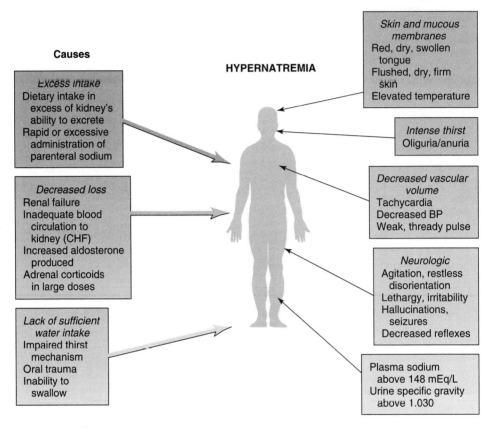

FIGURE 4-3

Causes and effects of hypernatremia. From Beare PG, Myers JL: *Adult health nursing*, ed 3, St Louis, 1998, Mosby.

356. Hypernatremia rarely occurs because usually the fluid intake is increased when sodium is resorbed. The more common problem with sodium excess is an increased ECF volume that results in edema.

increase

    Sodium excess is likely to cause an (increase, decrease) in ECF volume.

357. The symptoms will depend on the location of the edema. Edema of the lungs is called pulmonary edema and can occur in congestive heart failure. Edema location may vary; it is important to have a baseline assessment that identifies edematous areas to be able to detect the expansion or new onset of edematous areas.

vary

    Edematous areas may ____ from patient to patient.

358. If the edema is in the abdominal cavity, as occurs with
congestive heart failure or cirrhosis of the liver, the symptoms will result from the condition causing the ascites and
the pressure caused by the fluid. Edema in any tissue will
interfere with the nutrition of cells because blood flow is
limited to those cells.

   Whenever there is edema, the cells do not have good
nutrition, because blood flow is (increased, decreased) to   decreased
that part.

Treatment

359. The treatment of hypernatremia accompanied by increased
retention of water is aimed at the cause that produced the
excess. For example, in the person with pulmonary edema
caused by congestive heart failure, the treatment is aimed
at strengthening the contractions of the heart.

   The aim of treatment is to improve or correct the condition that caused _____ and _____ retention.   sodium
                                                                    water

   Another aspect of treatment is restriction of the intake
of sodium. The degree of restriction will vary. For some
persons, omitting salt in cooking will be an adequate restriction. For others, avoiding all salts or sodium such as
sodium chloride, sodium lactate, and sodium bicarbonate
may be necessary. There may be any degree of restriction
between these two extremes. If salt or sodium is restricted,
the nurse should be sure the patient understands the reasons for the restriction. The patient and the family must be
taught how to prepare food according to the restrictions.

   At times the intake of water is also restricted. If water is restricted, a schedule should be worked out so that the water or
fluid allowed is spaced over 24 hours. Because most people
sleep between the hours of 11 PM and 6 AM, patients should be
taught to create a fluid schedule that allows for the largest percentage of fluid to be taken during waking hours and the least
amount during the time they generally sleep. Some patients
wake during the night so restricting the fluid completely during
the sleep time hours may be a problem.

360. In treating edema caused by retention of sodium and water, the intake of _____ and _____ may be limited.   sodium
                                                                    water

361. Treatment may involve the use of diuretics, drugs that
prevent the resorption of sodium and water.

   Diuretics used to treat increased retention of sodium
and water act by _____ of sodium and wa-   preventing resorption
ter by the kidneys.

362. When diuretics are used, the nurse is responsible for keeping an accurate record of intake, output, and daily weight. This information is useful in avoiding overtreatment. It is possible to produce too great a loss of water and sodium as well as other electrolytes, especially potassium.

When diuretics are used, the nurse should record the following:

intake   a. _____

output   b. _____

daily weight   c. _____

363. If the increased resorption of sodium and water is caused by the overproduction of aldosterone, an antagonist, spironolactone (Aldactone), may be used.

aldosterone   Spironolactone is an antagonist to _____.

364. The treatment of sodium and water retention will depend on the cause but may include restricting sodium and water intake and the use of diuretics.

restricting   Treatment may include _____ sodium and water intake.

✓CONCEPT CHECK

In a healthy person the kidneys regulate the level of sodium. Certain hormonal or hemodynamic factors may cause the kidneys to be unable to maintain this balance. The conditions under which sodium excess (hypernatremia) may be a problem include renal failure with salt retention, inadequate blood flow to the kidneys (as in congestive heart failure), cirrhosis of the liver, overproduction of aldosterone by the adrenal glands, treatment with large doses of adrenal corticoids, or ingestion of greater than needed amounts of foods and fluids with a high sodium content.

Usually, when sodium is retained, water intake and/or resorption occurs. Thus the concentration of extracellular sodium does not increase, but rather there is an increase in ECF volume. The symptoms of this increase depend on the cause and the location of the edema. Treatment may include restriction of sodium and water intake and the use of diuretics.

✓INFORMATION CHECK

aldosterone   1. An increase in the hormone _____ will cause an increased resorption of sodium.

2. Inadequate blood flow to the kidneys will stimulate the production of _____, which will increase the resorption of
   sodium.   aldosterone

3. When an increased amount of sodium is resorbed, the person is stimulated to _____ water.   take in (drink)

4. When diuretics are used, the nurse should record the following:
   a. _____   intake
   b. _____   output
   c. _____   daily weight

5. After several days of vomiting and diarrhea, a patient was
   admitted to the hospital. The following morning his temperature was 105° F, heart rate was 150 beats/min, and respirations were 42/min. The laboratory results indicated his
   serum sodium was 150 mEq/L.
   a. This serum sodium level of 150 mEq/L is (high, low).   high
   b. With this serum sodium level, you (would, would not) be   would
      concern about his mental status.
   c. Care for this patient (would, would not) include restric-   would
      tion of foods and/or liquids with a high sodium content.

POTASSIUM IMBALANCE

Potassium is the major cation in intracellular fluid. In the body,
98% of the potassium is in the ICF, whereas only 2% is in the
ECF. The small amount in the ECF accounts for how a loss or
gain in potassium can have a significant effect on cardiac,
skeletal, and neuromuscular functioning. Serum potassium
tends to rise slightly with increasing age, especially in healthy
elderly men. It is also important to realize that many treatments,
medications, and diseases have an impact on maintaining adequate potassium levels. Table 4-1 shows normal potassium levels in children. The normal serum potassium level in older children and adults is 3.5 to 5 mEq/L.

TABLE 4-1 POTASSIUM LEVELS IN CHILDREN		
Specimen	Age	Normal Value (mEq/L)
Serum/plasma	Infant	3.0 to 6.0
	Child	3.5 to 5.0

From Wong DL, et al: *Whaley & Wong's nursing care of infants and children*, ed 6, St Louis, 1999, Mosby.

potassium   365. a. The major cation inside the cell is _____.
                  b. The normal level for serum potassium in older children
3.5 to 5   and adults is _____ mEq/L.

         366. One of the functions of potassium is to maintain the vol-
              ume of fluid within the cell. Remember we have already
              discussed that sodium is important in maintaining cell
              size. Because sodium is the primary cation outside cells
              and potassium is the primary cation inside cells, both are
              significant in controlling the movement of fluid in and out
              of cells by osmosis.
sodium   a. The primary cation in the ECF is _____.
                b. Both sodium and potassium are essential in controlling
osmosis   the movement of fluid in and out of cells by _____.

REMEMBER: The significance of the sodium-potassium pump is that it moves sodium out of the cell and potassium into the cell.

         367. Potassium is important in maintaining the volume of fluid
              within the cell. It is also necessary for the transmission of
              electrochemical impulses along the membranes of nerve
              and muscle cells. Therefore potassium is essential in reg-
              ulating neuromuscular irritability. This is particularly im-
              portant for the cardiac and skeletal muscle activity. Potas-
              sium easily diffuses through the cell membrane and
              moves positive electrical charges from inside the cell to
              outside the cell.
a cation   a. Potassium is (a cation, an anion).
positive   b. Therefore potassium carries a (positive, negative) elec-
                   trical charge.
                c. Potassium is necessary for the control of electrical im-
nerve   pulses in _____ and _____ cells.
muscle

         368. So far we have seen that potassium is important for the
              control of fluid volume within the cell and for regulating
              neuromuscular irritability. Another function of potassium
              is to control the hydrogen ion concentration (affecting
              acid-base balance). When potassium ions move out of the
              cell, sodium and hydrogen ions move into the cell.
cation   a. When one cation moves out of the cell, another _____
                   moves in to take its place.
sodium   b. As potassium ions move out of the cell, _____ and
hydrogen   _____ ions move into the cell.

         369. Potassium is important in controlling intracellular fluid
              volume, neuromuscular irritability, and hydrogen ion

concentration. The clinical signs and symptoms of potassium imbalance result primarily from altered neuromuscular irritability.

Three functions of potassium are the regulation of the following:

a. _____   intracellular fluid volume

b. _____   neuromuscular irritability

c. _____ H^+ concentration

370. Normally potassium is ingested in the diet. Because it is present in many foods, a person who is eating a diet that is adequate in calories and protein will likely have an adequate intake of potassium. About 80% of all the potassium that is ingested is excreted by the kidneys. The remaining 20% is excreted through the feces or sweat.

a. Potassium normally enters the body in the form of

_____.   food (diet)

b. About 80% of the potassium intake is excreted in the

_____.   urine

371. Although the filtered potassium is resorbed in the proximal tubules, the regulated excretion of potassium occurs in the distal tubules. The variations in excretion of potassium involve changes in potassium secretion and/or further potassium resorption. This regulation of potassium excretion is related to several other processes, which include sodium resorption, hydrogen ion excretion, and aldosterone level. For potassium to be excreted, adequate amounts of sodium must be available for exchange. When there is an increase in hydrogen ion excretion, there is a decrease in potassium excretion. An increased level of aldosterone stimulates an increased excretion of potassium.

Which of the following stimulates an increased excretion of potassium?

_____ a. Sodium deficit
_____ b. Decreased excretion of hydrogen ions   b
_____ c. Increased level of aldosterone   c
_____ d. Acidosis

372. When body fluids become too alkaline, the kidneys preserve hydrogen ions and excrete more potassium ions in exchange. Thus with alkalosis, large amounts of potassium may be excreted in the urine.

When alkalosis exists, (more, less) potassium is excreted in the urine.   more

373. The feedback mechanism of aldosterone in regulating potassium excretion is exactly opposite that for sodium regulation. When extracellular sodium concentration is low, aldosterone secretion is increased and more sodium is resorbed. When the extracellular level of potassium is high, more aldosterone is secreted and more potassium is excreted.

    When the production of aldosterone is stimulated, sodium is retained in the body and potassium is _____.

excreted

POTASSIUM DEFICIT (HYPOKALEMIA)

374. We have considered the function of potassium and the mechanisms for its control. We shall now look at the problem of a potassium deficit. Hypopotassemia, called **hypokalemia** (from the Latin word for potassium, "kalium"), is a low serum (ECF) potassium level less than 3.5 mEq/L.

hypokalemia
alkalosis

    A low serum level of potassium is called _____ or _____.

REMEMBER: Clinically we cannot measure the intracellular potassium.

Causes

375. We cannot conserve potassium. A low serum potassium level may occur when there is an inadequate intake or an increase in the excretion of potassium. Another cause is the presence of alkalosis. In alkalosis the serum potassium level may be low even though there is no loss of total body potassium.

alkalosis

    In (acidosis, alkalosis) the serum potassium level may be low even though the total body potassium level is normal.

Potassium

    _____ cannot be conserved.

376. Potassium loss causes a metabolic alkalosis, and the reverse is also true. A metabolic or respiratory alkalosis causes hypokalemia.

hypokalemia

    Alkalosis causes and can be caused by _____.

377. When potassium ions are lost from cells, sodium and hydrogen ions move into the cells to replace the potassium. Therefore the hydrogen ion concentration is decreased in the ECF and metabolic alkalosis results.

alkalosis

    Hypokalemia leads to metabolic (acidosis, alkalosis).

378. We shall now consider some of the causes of hy-
     pokalemia. Hypokalemia may be caused by (increased,   decreased
     decreased) intake and/or by _____ loss.   increased

REMEMBER: Hypokalemia is caused by either a decreased intake or an increased
loss of potassium.

Since normal kidneys continue to excrete some potassium,
the body must replace it. Normally the intake of potassium is
adequate in food and fluids. Even with an adequate intake of
potassium, hypokalemia may occur if there is excessive loss of
potassium. One way potassium may be lost is through the GI
tract. Vomiting, gastric suction, intestinal fistulas, or diarrhea
can cause a severe potassium loss.

When a patient loses an excessive amount of potassium from
the GI tract or from excessive sweating or because of being unable to eat a normal diet, potassium must be given by medication orally or via intravenous fluids. Additionally, patients who
are taking medication that waste potassium stores run the risk
of experiencing hypokalemia.

379. a. In a patient who is unable to eat a normal or adequate
        diet, supplements of potassium (will, will not) be nec-   will
        essary.
     b. Excessive potassium loss through either the GI tract or
        skin (may, may not) be responsible for hypokalemia.   may

380. A serious depletion of potassium can occur when GI se-
     cretions are lost through the following:
     a. _____   vomiting
     b. _____   gastric suction
     c. _____   intestinal fistulas
     d. _____   diarrhea

381. Hypokalemia may occur through loss of fluids from the GI
     tract. Loss of potassium also may occur through the uri-
     nary tract in several conditions. A high sodium intake or
     excessive administration of bicarbonate or other alkaline
     substances will stimulate the urinary loss of potassium.

     More potassium will be lost in the urine if the intake of
     sodium is (high, low).   high

382. Certain diseases of the kidneys that lead to potassium-
     losing nephritis can be another cause of hypokalemia, and
     potassium can be lost in the urine as a result of treatment

with diuretics. The thiazides and furosemide (Lasix) in particular cause loss of potassium. The very young and the very old are more likely to experience hypokalemia while taking any of the medications mentioned above.

hypo-

Use of furosemide or thiazide diuretics may result in (hyper-, hypo-) kalemia.

383. Use of adrenal cortical steroid hormones will increase the excretion of potassium. Earlier we learned that increased levels of aldosterone will stimulate the excretion of potassium. Therefore overproduction of adrenal cortical hormones or prolonged treatment with steroid drugs will cause loss of potassium.

increased

An increase in adrenal cortical steroid hormones will cause (increased, decreased) excretion of potassium.

384. We have seen that hypokalemia may be caused by inadequate intake or by increased loss of potassium. Elderly persons and/or any individual with previous health problems are at greater risk for developing hypokalemia related to a dietary insufficiency, the continued use of diuretics and laxatives, or the occurrence of diarrhea or inadequate renal function.

diarrhea

Potassium loss may occur through the GI tract with vomiting, gastric suction, intestinal fistulas, or _____.

385. In summation, increased amounts of potassium may be lost through the urinary tract in certain kidney diseases, with the use of certain diuretics, or with increased amounts of adrenal cortical steroid hormones (such as cortisone preparations) or with significant loss through the GI tract or skin.

Hypokalemia may occur because of increased urinary excretion of potassium from the following causes:

kidney disease   a. _____
certain diuretics   b. _____
adrenal cortical   c. _____
hormones

Signs and Symptoms

386. The nurse will assess for signs and symptoms of low potassium in persons who are likely to develop a deficit. The clinical signs and symptoms of potassium depletion may be evidenced by neuromuscular signs that include diminished deep tendon reflexes, muscular cramps, paresthesias, muscular weakness progressing to flaccid paralysis, fatigue, and mental confusion (Figure 4-4).

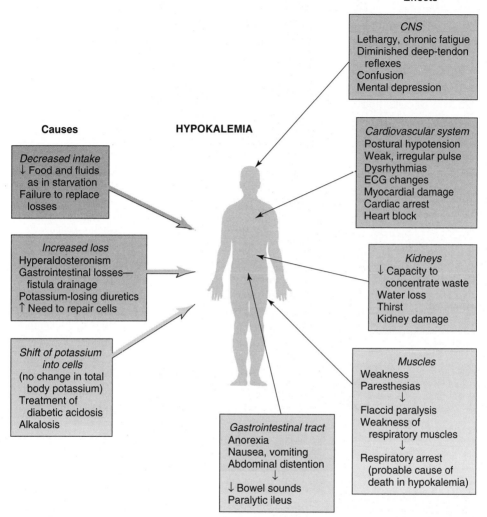

Effects

CNS
Lethargy, chronic fatigue
Diminished deep-tendon
  reflexes
Confusion
Mental depression

Causes   **HYPOKALEMIA**

Decreased intake
↓ Food and fluids
  as in starvation
Failure to replace
  losses

Cardiovascular system
Postural hypotension
Weak, irregular pulse
Dysrhythmias
ECG changes
Myocardial damage
Cardiac arrest
Heart block

Increased loss
Hyperaldosteronism
Gastrointestinal losses—
  fistula drainage
Potassium-losing diuretics
↑ Need to repair cells

Kidneys
↓ Capacity to
  concentrate waste
Water loss
Thirst
Kidney damage

*Shift of potassium
  into cells*
(no change in total
  body potassium)
Treatment of
  diabetic acidosis
Alkalosis

Muscles
Weakness
Paresthesias
  ↓
Flaccid paralysis
Weakness of
  respiratory muscles
  ↓
Respiratory arrest
  (probable cause of
  death in hypokalemia)

Gastrointestinal tract
Anorexia
Nausea, vomiting
Abdominal distention
  ↓
↓ Bowel sounds
Paralytic ileus

FIGURE **4-4**
Causes and effects of hypokalemia. From Beare PG, Myers JL: *Adult health nursing*, ed
3, St Louis, 1998, Mosby.

The neuromuscular signs of hypokalemia include the
following:
a. Paresthesias and muscle _____   cramps
b. Muscular weakness that may progress to _____   flaccid paralysis
_____
c. Fatigue and mental (alertness, confusion)   confusion

387. The GI signs of hypokalemia result from a reduction of neuromuscular irritability and a weakness of the smooth muscles of the GI tract. A low level of potassium in the body may cause anorexia, abdominal distention, and paralytic ileus (from an absent peristalsis).

Hypokalemia may cause the following GI signs:

anorexia   a. _____

abdominal distention   b. _____

paralytic ileus   c. _____

388. The most critical abnormality of renal function when the level of potassium in the body is low is the inability of the kidneys to concentrate urine. Therefore the quantity of urine is increased.

When the level of potassium in the body is low, the

increased   output of urine is (increased, unaffected, decreased).

389. Extreme depletion of potassium will involve the respiratory muscles. The diaphragm may be paralyzed. Respirations will become shallow, and death may result from apnea and respiratory arrest.

shallow   A severe deficit in potassium will cause (shallow, deep) respirations.

390. The cardiac signs of hypokalemia include irregular rhythm, heart block, altered electrocardiograph (ECG) patterns, myocardial damage, hypotension, and systolic arrest.

Hypokalemia may cause the following:

irregular   a. Cardiac signs that include a (regular, irregular) rhythm

Abnormal   b. (Normal, Abnormal) ECG patterns

arrest   c. Myocardial damage, hypotension, and systolic _____

391. A deficit in potassium will affect repolarization, which is evident on the ECG. In general, the ECG changes include a shortened and depressed S-T segment, a flattened or inverted T wave, a prolonged Q-T interval, and a U wave that is equal to or higher than the T wave.

flat   a. In hypokalemia the T wave is (flat, peaked).

lengthened   b. The Q-T interval is (shortened, lengthened).

present   c. A U wave is (present, absent).

Laboratory Findings

392. The normal serum potassium level varies from 3.5 to 5 mEq/L in adults (Table 4-2). The range is slightly nar-

TABLE 4-2	NORMAL LABORATORY VALUES OF ELECTROLYTES	
	Elements	Values
	Sodium	135–145 mEq/L
	Potassium	3.5–5.0 mEq/L
	Magnesium	1.5–2.5 mEq/L
	Calcium	4.5–5.0 mEq/L (ionized)
		8.5–10.5 mg/dl
	Phosphorus	2.5–4.5 mg/dl
	Chloride	95–108 mEq/L
	Bicarbonate	22–26 mEq/L

rower in children (see Table 4-1). When the serum potassium level is 3 mEq/L or lower, signs of hypokalemia may become evident.

a. Normal serum potassium levels in adults vary between
   ___ and _ mEq/L.   3.5, 5

b. Signs of hypokalemia may occur when the serum
   potassium level is _ mEq/L or lower.   3

REMEMBER: While conserving potassium in hypokalemia, the kidneys also increase the excretion of hydrogen ions, which causes alkalosis.

393. If the hypokalemia is severe, laboratory tests will indicate metabolic alkalosis.

    In severe hypokalemia the laboratory tests will indicate metabolic (acidosis, alkalosis).   alkalosis

394. A deficit in potassium enhances the action of digitalis. Therefore if digitalis is given to a person with hypokalemia, digitalis toxicity is more likely to occur.

    A toxic reaction to digitalis is more likely to occur if the potassium level is (high, normal, low).   low

Treatment
Treatment of hypokalemia is aimed at replacing the potassium that has been lost. Potassium can be given intravenously as a continous infusion or as a piggyback solution to achieve a quick response. **Potassium MAY NOT be given as a direct IV push; given IV push it is FATAL**.

395. The reason that potassium-containing solutions should not be given too rapidly intravenously is that the heart

muscle is very sensitive to extracellular potassium. If the concentration of potassium rises too rapidly, cardiac arrest may occur. When potassium is administered intravenously, the patient must be observed for symptoms of hyperkalemia.

If intravenous potassium is administered too rapidly, death may occur from cardiac _____.

arrest

396. Potassium given orally is also effective. However, the most natural way to replace potassium is through a high-potassium diet. Many foods contain potassium. Fruit juices (especially orange juice), bananas, bouillon and meat broths, and potatoes are rich sources.

List some foods that are rich in potassium:

orange juice   a. _____

bananas   b. _____

bouillon   c. _____

meat broths   d. _____

potatoes   e. _____

397. If potassium is to be replaced by oral medication, there are several forms that may be used: potassium chloride, potassium citrate, potassium gluconate, or combinations of these. Potassium-containing medications must be administered with caution because hyperkalemia can result from excessive dosages. Oliguria is an important sign of toxicity when potassium supplements are given.

A sign to watch for when potassium medications are being administered is (increased, decreased) urinary output.

decreased

398. If potassium is given intravenously, the rate must be limited. Forty milliequivalents of potassium should be diluted in 1000 ml of intravenous fluid for an adult. When potassium is given intravenously to an adult, the rate of infusion should not exceed 10 mEq/hr. When potassium is given to a child through a peripheral vein, the concentration should not exceed 30 to 40 mEq/L. Potassium supplements for a child are usually calculated at approximately 2 to 4 mEq/kg/24 hr.

a. When potassium chloride is given intravenously to an adult, it must be diluted and given at a rate of not more than __ mEq of potassium per hour.

10

b. When potassium is given intravenously to a child, the usual dose is calculated according to the _____ of the child.

weight

CONCEPT CHECK

Potassium is the major cation in the intracellular fluid. It is necessary to maintain the volume of fluid within the cell, to regulate neuromuscular irritability, and to maintain the hydrogen ion concentration in the body. Normally potassium is ingested with the diet and excreted by the kidneys. Normal kidneys will continue to excrete potassium even with inadequate intake; however, the regulation of potassium excretion depends on the amount of sodium available for exchange, the number of hydrogen ions being excreted, and the aldosterone level.

Clinically we do not measure the intracellular potassium; therefore the serum potassium level that is measured may not represent accurately the total body potassium. A low serum potassium is associated with alkalosis. Hypokalemia may be caused by a decreased intake or an increased loss of potassium.

Depletion of potassium may occur when GI secretions are lost through vomiting, gastric suction, intestinal fistulas, or diarrhea. Certain diseases of the kidney, treatment with diuretics, or increased adrenal cortical steroid hormones also may cause hypokalemia.

The clinical signs and symptoms of hypokalemia are not specific but include neuromuscular signs of diminished deep-tendon reflexes, muscle cramps, paresthesias, muscular weakness progressing to paralysis, fatigue, and mental confusion. The GI signs of hypokalemia include anorexia, abdominal distention, and paralytic ileus. The kidneys are unable to concentrate urine. The respirations become shallow, and death may result from apnea and respiratory arrest. The cardiac signs include irregular rhythm, heart block, altered ECG patterns, circulatory failure, hypotension, and systolic arrest. The normal serum potassium level is 3.5 to 5 mEq/L in an adult and 3.4 to 4.7 mEq/L in a child. The treatment for hypokalemia is replacement of potassium.

INFORMATION CHECK

1. The major intracellular cation is _____.

potassium

2. The kidneys (will, will not) continue to excrete potassium even when the intake of potassium is low.

will

3. Depletion of potassium may occur when GI secretions are lost through any of the following:
   a. _____

vomiting

   b. _____

gastric suction

   c. _____

intestinal fistulas

   d. _____

diarrhea

are not   4. Clinical signs and symptoms of hypokalemia (are, are not) specific.

paralysis   5. One of the symptoms of hypokalemia is muscular weakness that may progress to _____.

3.5 to 5   6. The normal serum potassium level for adults is _____ mEq/L.

is not   7. The serum potassium level (is, is not) always an accurate picture of the total body potassium level.

8. Which of the following persons may lose potassium?
a   _____ a. A person taking a diuretic
b   _____ b. A person taking a laxative

POTASSIUM EXCESS (HYPERKALEMIA)

Causes

399. Because normally functioning kidneys excrete potassium, abnormal potassium accumulation does not occur often. However, hyperpotassemia (or **hyperkalemia**), a serum level greater than 5.0 mEq/L, is extremely dangerous and can occur from excessive parenteral administration or overly rapid administration of solutions containing potassium. Blood transfusion also can cause hyperkalemia as a consequence of damage to the RBCs. Damage can occur with manipulation of RBCs or because of aging of the RBC cells. Both Situations allow potassium to escape into the ECF.

does not occur   a. Hyperkalemia (occurs, does not occur) frequently.
b. Excessive parenteral administration of potassium can
hyper-   cause (hyper-, hypo-) kalemia.

400. Trauma to tissues (such as crush injuries) will liberate intracellular potassium and result in hyperkalemia.
Intracellular potassium may be liberated by tissue
crush   trauma such as occurs in _____ injuries.

401. Adrenal cortical insufficiency will cause hyperkalemia. For example, in Addison's disease, in which aldosterone is lacking, potassium is not excreted normally. Therefore the level of potassium in the body goes up.
insufficiency   Adrenal cortical (insufficiency, overactivity) will cause hyperkalemia.

402. Respiratory or metabolic acidosis may cause the serum potassium level to rise. In acidosis the hydrogen ion concentration in the ECF increases. This causes potassium to move out of the cells; then hydrogen and sodium ions move into the cell. Therefore the level of potassium in the serum increases.
    a. Acidosis may cause (hypo-, hyper-) kalemia.   hyper-
    b. Alkalosis may cause (hypo-, hyper-) kalemia.   hypo-

403. In a patient with renal failure, the serum level of potassium may be difficult to control. Hyperkalemia is more likely to occur after the urinary output falls and urine and thus potassium is retained.

    In renal failure with a decreased urinary output, (hyper-, hypo-) kalemia may occur.   hyper-

404. Some of the more common causes of hyperkalemia include excessive administration of potassium, tissue trauma that liberates intracellular potassium, adrenal cortical insufficiency, acidosis, and renal failure with decreased urinary output. The major danger of hyperkalemia is its effect on the myocardium.

    The danger of hyperkalemia is the effect on the ____   heart (myocardium)
    _____.

405. Hyperkalemia is a medical emergency because of its effect on the heart. The danger is that the patient will die of cardiac standstill from a significantly elevated serum potassium. When complete heart block is associated with hyperkalemia, the rate may be slow, and the heart is in danger of stopping in diastole (Figure 4-5).
    a. Normal serum potassium in adults is _____ mEq/L.   3.5 to 5
    b. Heart block or ventricular standstill may occur when the _____ is significantly elevated.   potassium level

Signs and Symptoms
406. Neuromuscular symptoms of hyperkalemia include weakness that may progress to flaccid paralysis. Respiratory paralysis and involvement of the muscles of phonation may occur. Both hypokalemia and severe hyperkalemia may cause muscle paralysis. Movement of potassium and sodium is necessary for polarization and the spread of stimuli along the muscle fibers. If either persistent increased or decreased polarization occurs, the spread of the stimuli is blocked along the muscle fibers and muscle weakness or paralysis follows.

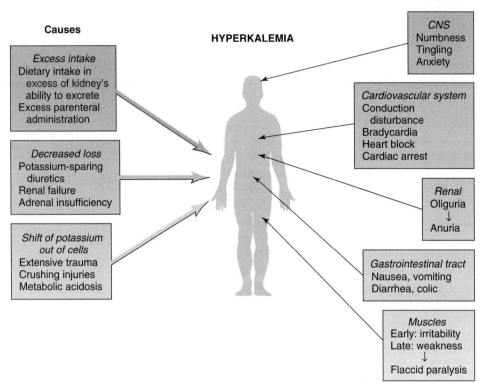

Causes

Excess intake
Dietary intake in
  excess of kidney's
  ability to excrete
Excess parenteral
  administration

Decreased loss
Potassium-sparing
  diuretics
Renal failure
Adrenal insufficiency

*Shift of potassium
  out of cells*
Extensive trauma
Crushing injuries
Metabolic acidosis

HYPERKALEMIA

Effects

CNS
Numbness
Tingling
Anxiety

Cardiovascular system
Conduction
  disturbance
Bradycardia
Heart block
Cardiac arrest

Renal
Oliguria
↓
Anuria

Gastrointestinal tract
Nausea, vomiting
Diarrhea, colic

Muscles
Early: irritability
Late: weakness
↓
Flaccid paralysis

FIGURE **4-5**
Causes and effects of hyperkalemia. From Beare PG, Myers JL: *Adult health nursing*, ed 3, St Louis, 1998, Mosby.

both hypo- and hyper-

Muscle weakness or paralysis is a symptom of (hypo-, hyper-, both hypo- and hyper-) kalemia.

Although potassium-sparing diuretics are more likely to cause hyperkalemia in older adults or any individuals whose health is compromised, hypokalemia is likely to occur whenever certain diuretics are used, even though they may be necessary to treat sodium and fluid volume excess.

407. Both hypokalemia and hyperkalemia may cause nausea, vomiting, muscle weakness, and paralysis. Paresthesias, or numbness and tingling sensations, are common in hyperkalemia.

hyper-

Paresthesias of the face, tongue, hands, and feet may be the result of (hypo-, hyper-) kalemia.

408. ECG changes in hyperkalemia include tall peaked T waves, widening of the QRS complex, and shortening of the Q-T interval. This is just the reverse of the ECG changes that occur in hypokalemia. Later the P-R interval becomes prolonged, and then the P waves flatten or disappear.

   ECG changes that occur in hyperkalemia include the following:
   a. T waves are _____.   tall and peaked
   b. Q-T interval is (shortened, lengthened).   shortened
   c. The _ wave disappears.   P

Laboratory Findings

409. The laboratory findings in hyperkalemia include a serum potassium of 6 mEq/L or higher.
   a. The normal serum potassium level is _____ mEq/L in   3.5 to 5
      adults.
   b. Serum potassium levels of _ mEq/L or higher are pres-   6
      ent in hyperkalemia.

410. Other laboratory findings are respiratory or metabolic acidosis. Hyperkalemia occurs in both respiratory and metabolic acidosis and is probably a compensatory mechanism. In acidosis the hydrogen ion concentration of the ECF increases, and, as the hydrogen and sodium ions move into the cell, they push potassium out into the ECF.

   In hyperkalemia, laboratory findings of respiratory or metabolic (acidosis, alkalosis) may be present.   acidosis

Treatment

411. The aim of treatment is to find the cause and correct it when possible. The method used to treat hyperkalemia will depend on the cause and severity of the hyperkalemia and on the patient's homeostatic mechanisms. An uncomplicated excess of potassium can be treated by avoiding additional potassium intake either orally or parenterally. A serum potassium level of 6.5 mEq/L and an abnormal ECG are considered an emergency. The immediate treatment is aimed at inducing potassium to enter the cells. Hypertonic glucose may be given intravenously to help potassium shift from the ECF to the liver and muscle cells.
   a. A serum potassium level of ___ mEq/L with an abnor-   6.5
      mal ECG is considered an emergency.
   b. Hypertonic glucose is given to help potassium move
      (into, out of) cells.   into

move into the cell

412. Insulin is given with the glucose to induce the movement of potassium back into the cells. Sodium bicarbonate may be used to buffer the hydrogen ion and allow the potassium to return to the cells.

The use of glucose, insulin, and sodium bicarbonate is aimed at helping the potassium to _____.

cells

413. Calcium gluconate may be administered intravenously in the treatment of hyperkalemia to increase the movement of potassium ions into tissue cells. Testosterone may be administered to prevent excessive protein breakdown and facilitate diffusion of potassium into bone and tissue cells.

Both calcium gluconate and testosterone are useful in making possible the movement of potassium from the ECF into the ____.

GI

414. Drugs such as cation-exchange resins may be used to remove potassium from the body through the GI tract. The cation-exchange resin, which is of the carboxylic acid type, gives up hydrogen ions for cations (for example, potassium, sodium, calcium). The resin can be given orally or rectally. The resins may cause constipation or impaction, and a mild laxative may be necessary.

Cation-exchange resins may be used in the treatment of hyperkalemia and act to remove potassium by way of the __ tract.

peritoneal dialysis or hemodialysis

415. If these measures are not successful in lowering the serum potassium level or if there is renal failure, the hyperkalemia should be treated by peritoneal dialysis or hemodialysis.

Hyperkalemia caused by renal failure should be treated by _____.

CONCEPT CHECK

Hyperkalemia does not occur often because normal kidneys continue to excrete potassium even when intake is not adequate. However, when it does occur, it may be caused by excessive parenteral administration of potassium, crush injuries, adrenal cortical insufficiency, and respiratory or metabolic acidosis. Another possible cause is renal failure with oliguria (decreased urinary output). The signs and symptoms of hyperkalemia are similar to those of hypokalemia except for the greater effect of hyperkalemia on the heart muscle.

Heart block and ventricular standstill may occur if the extracellular potassium is excessive. Muscle weakness and paralysis are symptoms of both hypokalemia and hyperkalemia. Paresthesias caused by hyperkalemia usually affect the face, tongue, hands, and feet.

In hyperkalemia the ECG changes include tall peaked T waves, widening of the QRS complex, and a shortened Q-T interval. The P-R interval becomes prolonged, and then the P waves flatten or disappear. A serum potassium level of 5 mEq/L or more is present in hyperkalemia. The immediate treatment is aimed at inducing potassium to enter the cells.

✓ INFORMATION CHECK

1. _____ may be caused by excessive administration of potassium.

    Hyperkalemia

2. Crush injuries and adrenal cortical (insufficiency, overactivity) may cause hyperkalemia.

    insufficiency

3. Hyperkalemia may be caused by respiratory or metabolic (acidosis, alkalosis).

    acidosis

4. In a person with renal failure, hyperkalemia is more likely to occur when the urinary output is (high, low).

    low

5. A serum potassium level of __ mEq/L or more is present in hyperkalemia.

    6

6. Mrs. Harvey has been admitted to the hospital complaining of increasing weakness. She has had gastritis for the last 3 days. Today she has been having muscle cramps and had difficulty getting out of bed.

    When her electrolyte report comes from the laboratory, you find the following: sodium, 139 mEq/L; potassium, 1 mEq/L; chloride, 96 mEq/L.

    a. Which of the electrolytes is the most abnormal? _____

    potassium

    b. With a very low potassium you would expect to find muscular _____.

    weakness

    c. The most likely cause for Mrs. Harvey's inability to get out of bed is _____.

    low potassium

    d. You learn that her feet had been swelling and the physician had given her diuretic pills, furosemide (Lasix), 2 weeks ago with the instruction to take one pill per day.

Recently the swelling did not go down overnight, so Mrs. Harvey began taking several extra Lasix tablets to reduce the swelling.

excretion

The explanation for Mrs. Harvey's weakness is the low potassium caused by urinary (excretion, retention) caused by taking the Lasix without an adequate intake of potassium.

e. With the data available, a possible nursing diagnosis could be: Knowledge deficit related to appropriate use of medication (Lasix) used for swelling of ankles as evidenced by muscle weakness and low serum potassium.

medication
signs, symptoms

Mrs. Harvey needs information about her _____, _____, and _____.

MAGNESIUM IMBALANCE

416. Magnesium is the fourth most abundant cation in the body. Like potassium, most of the magnesium is intracellular. Therefore only small amounts of magnesium are present in serum.

intracellular

a. Most of the magnesium in the body is in the (intravascular, intracellular, interstitial) compartment.

interstitial

b. The smallest amount of magnesium is in the (intravascular, intracellular, interstitial) compartment.

417. Approximately 60% of the total magnesium content of the body is present in bone. Only about 1% of the body's magnesium is in the ECF; the remaining magnesium is within the cells. The normal serum level of magnesium is 1.5 to 2.5 mEq/L in adults and 1.3 to 2.4 mEq/L in infants. The magnesium level may be slightly lower in the elderly than in younger adults.

a. The percentage of magnesium that is extracellular is

1%

___.

1.5, 2.5

b. The normal serum magnesium is __ to __ mEq/L in adults.

418. Magnesium has several essential functions. Magnesium has been recognized more recently as being more crucial to body function than some other electrolytes. Magnesium functions as an activator in many enzyme reactions. Some of the enzyme systems that magnesium activates are those that empower the B vitamins to function and those that are associated with carbohydrate and protein metabolism. Magnesium assists in the production and use

of adenosine triphosphate (ATP), which serves as the energy source for the sodium-potassium pump and is required for the synthesis of nucleic acids and proteins.

a. Magnesium is necessary as an activator of many _____ systems.

b. The synthesis of nucleic acid and proteins requires _____.

enzyme

magnesium

419. Another function of magnesium is that it exerts an effect similar to that of calcium on neuromuscular function. At some points magnesium acts synergistically with calcium, whereas at others it is antagonistic. Magnesium affects skeletal muscle directly by depressing acetylcholine release at the synaptic junction. Therefore neuromuscular activity is increased when magnesium levels are decreased. Magnesium is commonly used to prevent convulsions in toxemia of pregnancy.

When magnesium levels are increased, neuromuscular activity is (increased, decreased).

decreased

420. So far we have seen that magnesium is essential as an activator in many enzyme reactions. It is especially necessary for carbohydrate metabolism, and it is required for the synthesis of nucleic acids and proteins. Magnesium affects neuromuscular functions; it also facilitates the transportation of sodium and potassium across cell membranes. If magnesium is deficient, the kidneys tend to excrete more potassium.

When magnesium is deficient, the kidneys are likely to excrete (more, less) potassium.

more

421. Magnesium effects parathyroid hormone secretion and therefore influences the levels of intracellular calcium. If the level of magnesium in the body is below normal, the action of parathyroid hormone in maintaining normal serum calcium levels is impaired.

Magnesium influences the level of intracellular calcium by its effect on the secretion of _____ _____.

parathyroid hormone

422. Finally, magnesium affects the irritability and contractility of cardiac muscle and influences vasodilation and cardiac output.

Magnesium level (does, does not) affect cardiac functioning

does

423. Magnesium therefore functions as an activator in many enzyme reactions, in carbohydrate and protein metabolism, in the synthesis of nucleic acids and proteins, in neuromuscular and cardiovascular function, and in the transportation of sodium and potassium across cell membranes as well as influencing the levels of intracellular calcium. A healthy adult ingests about 25 mEq of magnesium per day, of which about 40% is absorbed by the intestine. Recommended foods that are high in magnesium include unprocessed cereal grains (such as oats and bran), nuts, chocolate, green leafy vegetables and dry beans and peas (legumes).

nuts, legumes
chocolate
green leaf
vegetables
25

a. Foods that are high in magnesium include unprocessed cereal grains, ____, _____, _____, and _____ _____.

b. A healthy adult ingests approximately ___ mEq of magnesium per day.

Although unprocessed cereal grains (oats and bran), nuts, and legumes are good sources of magnesium, other foods contain magnesium as well. Vegetables and fruits such as bananas are good sources. Magnesium also is plentiful in meats, fish, and peanut butter.

424. Which of the following foods contain abundant amounts of magnesium?

a   _____ a. Broccoli
           _____ b. Milk
c   _____ c. Almonds
           _____ d. Honey
e   _____ e. Oat or bran cereals
f   _____ f. Chocolate

REMEMBER: Magnesium is absorbed from the intestine.

425. Magnesium is regulated by the intestine and kidneys. Physiologic factors that influence normal absorption include the total magnesium intake; the length of time it is in the intestine; the rate of water absorption; and the amounts of calcium, phosphate, and lactose in the diet. It is understandable that persons who have had intestinal bypass surgery for obesity may develop magnesium deficiency.

diet
intestine

a. Magnesium is usually taken into the body in the normal ____.

b. Magnesium is absorbed from the _____.

426. Magnesium is excreted from the body primarily in the urine. The kidneys are able to conserve magnesium ions, so renal excretion of magnesium may be less than 1 mEq/day on a magnesium-free diet, after a period of adjustment.
     a. The major pathway for magnesium loss is _____.   in the urine
     b. The kidneys (are, are not) able to conserve magnesium.   are

MAGNESIUM DEFICIT (HYPOMAGNESEMIA)

427. We have considered the function, as well as the intake and loss, of magnesium. Because most of the body's magnesium is inside the cells, identifying a person's actual serum level may be difficult. For instance, the significant link to albumin, in which a low albumin level will reflect a low magnesium level even if the magnesium is actually within normal limits, interferes with a true interpretation of laboratory results. When a low serum magnesium level does exist, it is called **hypomagnesemia**. Hypomagnesemia is present when the serum concentration of magnesium is less than 1.5 mEq/L.
     a. Normal serum magnesium in adults is __ to __ mEq/L.   1.5, 2.5
     b. Hypomagnesemia is present when the serum magnesium is less than __ mEq/L.   1.5

REMEMBER: Only 1% of the magnesium in the body is extracellular. Therefore there is no direct correlation between serum concentration and the total body store of magnesium.

---

428. Usually when symptoms are present, the serum magnesium concentration will be below 1 mEq/L.
         When symptoms of hypomagnesemia are present, the serum magnesium usually will be below _ mEq/L.   1

Causes

429. A deficit in magnesium is usually not the result of dietary restrictions. However, it can occur with prolonged malnutrition or starvation, or if a patient is given magnesium-free fluids intravenously along with no oral intake and/or with nasogastric suction. Persons receiving parenteral hyperalimentation (total parenteral nutrition) in which there is inadequate magnesium may develop hypomagnesemia (Figure 4-6).
     a. An inadequate intake of magnesium will lead to
        _____.   hypomagnesemia

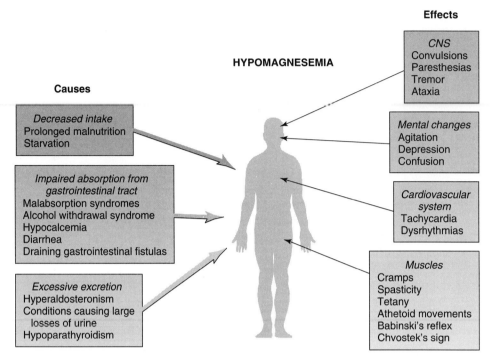

Effects

HYPOMAGNESEMIA

Causes

Decreased intake
Prolonged malnutrition
Starvation

Impaired absorption from gastrointestinal tract
Malabsorption syndromes
Alcohol withdrawal syndrome
Hypocalcemia
Diarrhea
Draining gastrointestinal fistulas

Excessive excretion
Hyperaldosteronism
Conditions causing large losses of urine
Hypoparathyroidism

CNS
Convulsions
Paresthesias
Tremor
Ataxia

Mental changes
Agitation
Depression
Confusion

Cardiovascular system
Tachycardia
Dysrhythmias

Muscles
Cramps
Spasticity
Tetany
Athetoid movements
Babinski's reflex
Chvostek's sign

FIGURE 4-6

Causes and effects of hypomagnesemia. From Beare PG, Myers JL: *Adult health nursing*, ed 3, St Louis, 1998, Mosby.

do

b. Persons who are receiving no oral intake (do, do not) need magnesium added to the intravenous fluids.

430. Hypomagnesemia can be caused by inadequate intake; however, a more common cause is impaired intestinal absorption.

Impaired intestinal absorption of magnesium will lead

hypomagnesemia   to _____.

431. Children or adults with malabsorption syndrome or chronic diarrhea may develop hypomagnesemia. Persons with GI fistulas also may develop hypomagnesemia. In these patients magnesium is excreted in the stool in the form of magnesium soaps.

Persons with malabsorption syndrome or chronic diar-

hypo-   rhea may develop (hyper-, hypo-) magnesemia.

432. Another cause of hypomagnesemia is an excessive intake of calcium, which impairs magnesium absorption be-

cause these two compounds compete for the same absorption site.

Hypomagnesemia may be caused by an excessive intake of _____.

calcium

433. Magnesium deficit can be induced by alcoholism. Alcohol ingestion seems to promote a magnesium deficit because of the related poor nutritional intake of magnesium and increased urinary secretion.

Alcohol ingestion seems to promote a magnesium (deficit, excess).

deficit

434. Other causes of impaired absorption of magnesium include bowel resection, small bowel bypass, inherited intestinal defects in magnesium absorption, or chronic irritable bowel disorders.

Bowel resection or diseases may contribute to a magnesium (deficit, excess).

deficit

435. We have considered inadequate intake of magnesium and impaired absorption of magnesium as causes of hypomagnesemia. Other causes of hypomagnesemia include excessive renal excretion or fluid loss.

Three categories of causes of hypomagnesemia include the following:
a. _____
b. _____
c. _____

inadequate intake
impaired absorption
excessive loss

436. The usual cause of excessive renal excretion of magnesium is diuretic therapy. Subsequently, individuals who are taking a combination of a diuretic and a cardiac glycoside such as digitalis are at greater risk of digitalis toxicity. A low magnesium level may lead to a retention of digoxin.

A common cause of excessive renal excretion of magnesium is _____ therapy.

diuretic

437. Another cause of hypomagnesemia is major surgery. After major surgery, excessive urinary loss of magnesium occurs for 24 hours.

During the first 24 hours after major surgery, excessive urinary (loss, retention) of magnesium occurs.

loss

438. Increased magnesium loss also occurs because of excessive urine excretion that occurs in diabetic ketoacidosis,

primary aldosteronism, primary hyperparathyroidism, and other hypercalcemic states.

increased

In diabetic ketoacidosis (increased, decreased) magnesium loss occurs.

439. Excessive urinary excretion of magnesium may occur with several types of renal disease.

magnesium

Renal disease may cause increased urinary excretion of _____.

440. In considering excessive renal loss of magnesium we have included diuretic therapy, major surgery, diabetic ketoacidosis, primary aldosteronism, primary hyperparathyroidism, and other hypercalcemic states as well as renal disease. Hypomagnesemia also may occur in hypoparathyroidism in association with hypocalcemia. Whenever hypocalcemia and hypokalemia exist, expect to find hypomagnesemia as well.

low

When a person has low calcium and low potassium levels, you should expect to find a (high, low) level of magnesium.

Signs and Symptoms

Certain signs and symptoms that are commonly seen with a magnesium deficit are generally linked to magnesium's effect on neuromuscular and cardiovascular function. The signs and symptoms of magnesium deficit that are characterized by neuromuscular irritability include tremor, athetoid or choreiform movements (slow, involuntary twisting and writhing movements), tetany, ataxia, increased reflexes, clonus, a positive Babinski's sign, a positive Chvostek's sign, paresthesias of the feet and legs, excessive neuromuscular irritability, and convulsions.

441. A positive Babinski's sign is dorsiflexion of the great toe with fanning of the other toes when the lateral aspect of the sole is stroked sharply (Figure 4-7). However, in an infant this is a normal response until about 2 years of age. Chvostek's sign is elicited by tapping the person's face just in front of the ear over the facial nerve. Tapping over the nerve will cause unilateral spasm of the lip, nose, or eyelid when the test is positive.

irritability

The signs and symptoms of magnesium deficit are characterized by neuromuscular _____.

442. Which of the following are signs or symptoms of magnesium deficit?

A   B

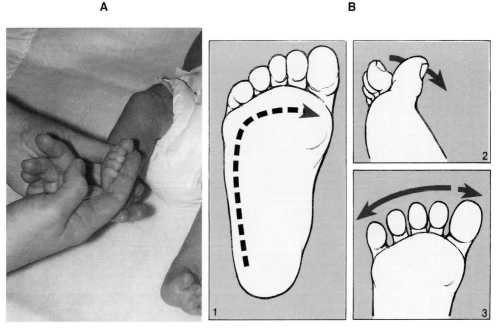

FIGURE **4-7**
A, Plantar or grasp reflex. **B**, Babinski's reflex. **A** from Zitelli BJ, Davis HW: *Atlas of pediatric physical diagnosis*, ed 3, St Louis, 1997, Mosby. **B** from Wong DL, et al: *Whaley & Wong's nursing care of infants and children*, ed 6, St Louis, 1999, Mosby.

_____ a. Tremor   a
_____ b. Negative Babinski's sign
_____ c. Tetany   c
_____ d. Increased reflexes   d
_____ e. Lethargy
_____ f. Convulsions   f

443. Other signs and symptoms of magnesium deficit include personality changes along with agitation, mental depression or confusion, and hallucinations, which are usually auditory or visual.

    A person who develops a personality change with agitation, becomes mentally depressed or confused, or develops hallucinations may have a magnesium (deficit, excess).   deficit

444. There may be cardiovascular signs and symptoms related to a magnesium deficit, including tachycardia with atrial or ventricular premature contractions, nonspecific T wave changes in the electrocardiogram, and ventricular fibrillation.

Which of the following signs may result from magnesium deficit?

_____ a. Bradycardia

b   _____ b. Atrial or ventricular premature contractions

c   _____ c. Nonspecific T wave changes

d   _____ d. Ventricular fibrillation

445. Most of the signs and symptoms of a magnesium deficit are related to the neuromuscular, neurologic, and cardiovascular systems. Hypomagnesemia and hypocalcemia may coexist. This is especially true in persons with an excessive loss of GI fluids.

neurologic
neuromuscular
cardiovascular
hypo-

a. Most of the signs and symptoms of a magnesium deficit are related to the _____, _____, and _____ systems.

b. When hypocalcemia is present, (hyper-, hypo-) magnesemia also may be present.

446. Hypomagnesemia and hypercalcemia also may coexist in persons with hyperparathyroidism and in persons who have neoplastic disease with osteolytic metastasis (metastasis to bone).

In persons with hyperparathyroid function or who have neoplastic disease with metastasis to bone, hypomagnesemia may coexist along with (hypo-, hyper-) calcemia.

hyper-

447. A deficit in magnesium may precipitate or aggravate digitalis toxicity.

A toxic reaction to digitalis is more likely to occur if the serum magnesium is (high, low).

low

Treatment

448. Treatment of hypomagnesemia consists of correcting the underlying cause of the low serum magnesium intravenously, intramuscularly, or orally with magnesium salts. Magnesium sulfate is the most commonly used magnesium salt.

correcting the cause

a. Hypomagnesemia should be treated by first _____
_____.

b. The most commonly used magnesium salt is

magnesium sulfate

_____.

449. Magnesium salts can be given orally to counteract continuous excessive losses. When magnesium is given orally, diarrhea is a possible side effect.

A possible side effect of magnesium salts given orally
is _____.

diarrhea

450. In an adult, magnesium sulfate can be given intramuscularly in a dose of 2 g (16.3 mEq) every 8 hours for 3 to 5
days. Repeated intramuscular injections should be given
at different sites because the injections may be painful.
Procaine hydrochloride 1% can be added to the injection
if a large dose is used.

Intramuscular injections of magnesium sulfate are
(likely, not likely) to be painful.

likely

451. In an adult, magnesium sulfate can also be given intravenously when hypomagnesemia is severe and may be associated with convulsions. When magnesium sulfate is
given intravenously in an emergency situation to an adult,
a loading dose of 500 mg of magnesium may be given at
an extremely slow rate (15 mg/min). It may be followed
by a continuous intravenous infusion of magnesium solution given slowly over 24 hours. This infusion must be
given through an infusion pump, and the patient must be
monitored closely.

In an emergency, the safe rate for giving magnesium
intravenously to an adult is __ mg/min.

15

452. During an intravenous infusion of magnesium sulfate, the
patient should not be left alone. You should observe the
effectiveness of the magnesium infusion in relieving signs
and symptoms. Observe for the anticonvulsant effect, re-
laxation of spastic muscles, and resolution of tremors and
arrhythmias.

Signs indicating that the magnesium infusion is effective include a decrease in the following symptoms:
a. _____
b. _____
c. _____

muscle tension
tremors
arrhythmias

453. Whenever magnesium sulfate is given intravenously, you
must monitor the patient for signs and symptoms of high
serum magnesium. Check every 5 minutes or before each
dose for flaccidity and loss of patellar (knee-jerk) reflex.
a. When giving magnesium sulfate intravenously, you
must monitor the patient for signs of (high, low) serum
magnesium.
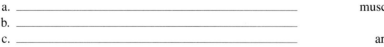
b. You should check for loss of patellar reflex every _____
minutes.

high

5

454. In addition to checking for loss of the patellar reflex, you should also count the respiratory rate every 5 minutes and place the patient on continuous cardiac monitoring. Be sure the respiratory rate is at least 16/min. Respiratory paralysis may occur during infusion of magnesium sulfate.

loss of patellar reflex

respiratory rate

During intravenous infusion of magnesium sulfate, you should check for _____ and _____ every 5 minutes.

455. During intravenous infusion of magnesium sulfate, you should look for flushing of the skin, especially of the face, and for diaphoresis.

redness

moist

Observations to be made during an intravenous infusion of magnesium sulfate include (redness, paleness) of the face and (moist, dry) skin.

456. In addition to checking reflexes, respiratory rate, and condition of the skin, you need to check the blood pressure of the person receiving magnesium sulfate intravenously. During an infusion, you should check the patient's blood pressure every 5 to 10 minutes to detect hypotension.

5, 10

During infusion of magnesium sulfate, the blood pressure should be checked every _ to _ minutes.

457. When giving intravenous infusion of magnesium sulfate, you should slow or stop the infusion and notify the physician if any one of the following signs appears: loss of the patellar reflex, decreased respiratory rate, flushing of the face, diaphoresis, flaccidity, or hypotension.

During intravenous infusion of magnesium sulfate, you should slow or stop the infusion if which of the following signs appear?

a

_____ a. Loss of the patellar reflex

_____ b. Increased respiratory rate of 24

c

_____ c. Flushing of the face

_____ d. Spasticity

e

_____ e. Hypotension

458. If magnesium levels become high, respiratory failure may occur.

failure

If magnesium levels become high, you must be prepared to manage respiratory _____.

459. One of the prime responsibilities of the nurse in caring for a person with a magnesium deficit is to provide for the pa-

tient's safety. Since convulsions may occur, protective measures must be taken to prevent injury.

Persons with a magnesium deficit must be protected from injury that could result during a _____.

convulsion

460. Another reason why persons with a magnesium deficit have special safety needs is that they may become confused and/or may develop hallucinations.

Persons with a magnesium deficit need to be protected because they may become (drowsy, confused) and may develop hallucinations.

confused

✓CONCEPT CHECK

Magnesium is the second most abundant cation in the intracellular fluid. Magnesium is essential as an activator in many enzyme reactions, especially carbohydrate metabolism. It is required for the synthesis of nucleic acids and proteins and is important for normal neuromuscular function. It influences the levels of intracellular calcium and facilitates transportation of sodium and potassium across cell membranes.

Most of the magnesium is in the intracellular fluid. Only about 1% of magnesium is extracellular. Normal serum magnesium is 1.5 to 2.5 mEq/L in adults and 1.3 to 2.4 mEq/L in infants.

Magnesium deficit may occur with prolonged malnutrition, starvation, alcoholism, or administration of magnesium-free intravenous fluids along with no oral intake. A deficit in magnesium may be caused by impaired intestinal absorption or loss through diarrhea or draining GI fistulas. Excessive loss of magnesium may occur through renal excretion.

The clinical signs and symptoms of hypomagnesemia are not specific but may include mental changes such as personality change, agitation, mental depression, confusion, or hallucinations. The neuromuscular signs and symptoms include tremor, tetany, clonus, increased reflexes, positive Babinski's sign, positive Chvostek's sign, paresthesias, and convulsions. The cardiovascular signs and symptoms include tachycardia, atrial or ventricular premature contractions, and nonspecific T wave or atrial fibrillation changes in the electrocardiogram.

✓INFORMATION CHECK

1. The second major intracellular cation is _____.

magnesium

2. Magnesium is essential as an activator in many _____ reactions.

enzyme

1.5, 2.5   3. Normal serum magnesium is ___ to ___ mEq/L in an adult.

4. A magnesium deficit may result from inadequate intake because of:

malnutrition or   a. _____
starvation
alcoholism   b. _____
magnesium-free   c. _____
intravenous fluids

5. Excessive loss of magnesium may be caused by intestinal conditions such as:

malabsorption   a. _____
diarrhea   b. _____
fistulas   c. _____

6. Clinical signs and symptoms of hypomagnesemia (are, are
are not   not) specific.

7. Personality change, confusion, or hallucinations may occur
hypo-   with (hypo-, hyper-) magnesemia.

8. Which of the following are neuromuscular signs and symptoms of hypomagnesemia?
a   _____ a. Tremor
   _____ b. Depressed reflexes
c   _____ c. Positive Babinski's sign
d   _____ d. Convulsions

MAGNESIUM EXCESS (HYPERMAGNESEMIA)

Causes

461. Magnesium excess, or **hypermagnesemia**, is not a common imbalance. Hypermagnesemia seldom develops except in renal failure and is generally caused by a decrease in excretion.

The most common cause of hypermagnesemia is ___
renal failure   ___.

462. Hypermagnesemia is a serum magnesium level over 2.5 mEq/L.
1.5, 2.5   a. Normal serum magnesium in adults is ___ to ___ mEq/L.
   b. A serum magnesium level of 3 mEq/L would be called
hypermagnesemia   _____.

463. Although renal failure is the most common cause of hypermagnesemia, excessive use of magnesium-containing medications can also contribute to hypermagnesemia. A person with renal failure who takes large amounts of magnesium-containing antacids or cathartics may develop hypermagnesemia.

A person, especially an individual with a history of renal failure, who takes large amounts of magnesium-containing antacids is at risk for (hyper-, hypo-) magnesemia.

hyper-

464. Hypermagnesemia occurs in a person with diabetic ketoacidosis when there has been severe water loss.

A person who has diabetic ketoacidosis with severe dehydration may develop _____.

hypermagnesemia

Signs and Symptoms

465. The signs and symptoms of hypermagnesemia will vary with the level of serum magnesium and are related to a depressed central nervous system (CNS). When the serum magnesium is between 3 and 5 mEq/L, the vasodilating effect of magnesium can cause hypotension. Flushing, a feeling of warmth, nausea, diminished deep reflexes, and diaphoresis may also occur.

A patient with a serum magnesium of _ to _ mEq/L may have hypotension.

3, 5

466. When serum magnesium increases to a level of 5 to 7 mEq/L, behaviors associated with hypermagnesemia become more pronounced. These include drowsiness, bradycardia, significant loss of deep tendon reflexes, and worsening hypotension.
   a. A person may become drowsy when the serum magnesium level is over _ mEq/L.

5

   b. When the serum magnesium level is 7 mEq/L, the deep tendon reflexes are (increased, decreased, absent).

absent

467. The respiratory center is depressed when the serum magnesium rises to greater than 7, and, as the magnesium increases, the respiratory compromise increases as well.

Respiratory depression occurs as the serum level of magnesium (increases, decreases).

increases

468. Coma, heart block, and respiratory arrest may occur at serum magnesium levels of 12 to 15 mEq/L, and cardiac arrest occurs at concentrations of 15 to 20 mEq/L.

cardiac

At serum magnesium levels over 15 mEq/L, coma is likely to occur, followed by _____ arrest.

469. The sequence of the signs and symptoms of increasing magnesemia are hypotension, drowsiness, loss of deep tendon reflexes, respiratory depression, coma, and cardiac arrest.

7

Loss of deep tendon reflexes is likely to occur at a serum magnesium level of _ mEq/L.

Treatment

470. Interventions are aimed at treating the cause of the magnesium excess. They range from increasing fluid intake to produce an increase in urinary output to dialysis to remove the increase in magnesium. Magnesium salts should not be given to persons with renal failure. If renal failure is present, dialysis will likely be necessary even though dialysis is not very efficient in removing magnesium.

should not

Persons with renal failure (should, should not) take medications containing magnesium salts.

471. Another useful treatment for hypermagnesemia is the use of intravenous calcium gluconate. Calcium has an antagonistic effect on magnesium and can therefore be a useful temporary measure.

An electrolyte that has an antagonistic effect on magnesium and may be used in treating hypermagnesemia is

calcium

_____.

The nurse must assess patients for signs and symptoms that would indicate possible increasing hypermagnesemia and those related to each level of hypermagnesemia. For example, monitor vital signs, cardiac and respiratory rate, and deep tendon reflexes. It is important that the nurse provide for the patient's safety because of the muscle weakness.

✓CONCEPT CHECK

Hypermagnesemia seldom occurs except in persons with renal failure or those with an increase in intake that causes an increase in output. A serum level of magnesium over 2.5 mEq/L is hypermagnesemia. Excessive use of magnesium-containing medications by a person with renal failure can contribute to hypermagnesemia. Persons with diabetic ketoacidosis and severe water loss may develop hypermagnesemia. The signs and symptoms of hypermagnesemia progress from hypotension, flushing, diaphoresis, drowsiness, loss of deep tendon reflexes, and respiratory depression to coma and cardiac arrest.

INFORMATION CHECK

1. A serum magnesium of 3 mEq/L is _____.

hypermagnesemia

2. The most common cause of hypermagnesemia is _____ _____.

renal failure

3. One of the earliest signs indicating hypermagnesemia is _____.

hypotension

4. At a serum magnesium level of 7 mEq/L, deep tendon reflexes are likely to be _____.

absent

5. Calcium gluconate is sometimes used in treating hypermagnesemia because calcium is _____ to magnesium.

antagonistic

CALCIUM IMBALANCE

472. Serum calcium imbalance can be a real medical emergency; therefore it is important for you to know how the body normally balances calcium and how to anticipate and recognize a calcium imbalance. Calcium is the most abundant cation in the body. However, 99% of the calcium is in the bones.

Calcium is the most abundant (cation, anion) in the body.

cation

473. The other 1% of the calcium in the body is in the blood plasma or serum. The calcium concentration in the extracellular compartment usually remains remarkably constant. Normally the total serum calcium is 8.5 to 10.5 mg/dl (4.5 to 5.0 mEq/L ionized).
    a. The amount of calcium in serum is _ %.

1

    b. Normally the serum calcium concentration (remains constant, fluctuates widely).

remains constant

474. Calcium in the intravascular compartment is mainly in two forms: one form is ionized calcium, which is physiologically active; the second form is calcium that is bound to protein, particularly albumin. The serum levels reported usually include both the protein and ionized forms.
    a. The form of calcium that is physiologically active is _____ calcium.

ionized

    b. The bound calcium in the blood is bound to _____.

protein

475. Normally 50% to 75% of the serum calcium is ionized.
     a. Ionized serum calcium is physiologically (inactive,
active   active).
50, 75   b. The amount of serum calcium that is ionized is __% to
        __%.

476. Although 50% to 75% of the serum calcium is ionized,
     the rest is bound to protein. Most of the bound calcium is
     combined with albumin. The calcium that is bound to
     plasma protein cannot pass through the capillary wall and
     therefore cannot leave the intravascular compartment. It
     is the ionized calcium that is involved in furtherance of
     neuromuscular activity.
     a. Most of the calcium that is bound to protein is bound
albumin   to _____.
cannot   b. Calcium that is bound to plasma protein (can, cannot)
        pass through the capillary wall.
is   c. Ionized calcium (is, is not) associated with the promo-
        tion of neuromuscular activity.

477. Clinically the serum calcium level can be misleading un-
     less it is correlated with the serum albumin level. As the
     total protein in the blood decreases, less serum calcium is
     bound.
     a. The serum calcium level should be correlated with the
albumin   serum _____ level.
     b. When the total protein in the blood decreases, (more,
less   less) calcium is bound.

478. Any change in serum protein will result in a change in the
     total serum calcium.
a decrease   A decrease in serum protein will result in (a decrease,
     an increase) in serum calcium.

479. One of the functions of calcium, along with phosphorus, is
     to provide strength and durability to bones and teeth. As we
     learned earlier, 99% of the calcium is in the bones. Even
     though the serum calcium is a small percentage of the total,
     it is essential for some vital physiologic processes.
strength   a. Calcium provides _____ and _____ to bones and
durability   teeth.
essential   b. The calcium in the serum is (essential, nonessential)
        for some of the vital physiologic processes.

480. Free, ionized calcium is needed to help maintain the per-
     meability of cell membranes. Calcium is essential for the

transmission of nerve impulses and neuromuscular excitability, and it is necessary for normal cardiac function.

a. Calcium is necessary to help maintain the _____ of cell membranes.

permeability

b. Calcium is necessary for the _____ of nerve impulses.

transmission

481. In addition to helping maintain the permeability of cell membranes and influencing neuromuscular function, calcium is needed for blood coagulation.

Calcium is (needed, not needed) for blood coagulation.

needed

482. Calcium is also important in activating enzyme reactions and hormone secretion.

Calcium functions by _____ enzyme reactions.

activating

483. Nerve cell membranes are less excitable when sufficient calcium is available.

Calcium acts as a (sedative, stimulant) on nerve cell membranes.

sedative

484. We have considered some of the functions of calcium. Our bodies have several ways to regulate the level of calcium in serum. Homeostasis of calcium occurs by the interchange of calcium ions moving in and out of the extracellular space. Hence, calcium enters the ECF through resorption of calcium ions from bone, absorption of dietary calcium in the GI tract, and from reabsorption of calcium from the kidneys.

List three sources of serum calcium:

a. _____

bone resorption

b. _____

intestinal absorption

c. _____

renal resorption

485. Serum calcium leaves the ECF through the process of bone deposition and as a result of renal and fecal excretion.

a. Serum calcium is decreased by bone (deposition, resorption).

deposition

b. Serum calcium is decreased by fecal (excretion, resorption).

excretion

c. Serum calcium is decreased by renal (resorption, excretion).

excretion

486. The serum calcium level is influenced by both the resorption and the formation of bone. Bone deposition or formation occurs in response to stress and strain.

deposition

Stress and strain on the skeleton results in bone (deposition, resorption).

487. The major factors that control the serum calcium concentration are vitamin D, parathyroid hormone, calcitonin (thyrocalcitonin), and serum concentrations of calcium and phosphate ions.

D

a. The vitamin that is important in controlling the serum calcium concentration is __.

parathyroid
calcitonin

b. The two hormones that are important in the control of serum calcium concentration are _____ and _____.

weak

c. Calcitonin has a (weak, strong) effect on the serum calcium concentration.

phosphate

d. Serum concentrations of calcium and _____ ions influence the serum calcium level.

488. Vitamin D, essential for regulating calcium, is ingested in food, particularly dairy products, or is synthesized in the body by the skin after being exposed to ultraviolet light. Two sources of vitamin D are:

food

a. _____

synthesis in the body

b. _____

489. The general actions of vitamin D are to increase serum calcium through absorption from the GI tract, the mobilization of calcium ions from the bones through resorption, and by kidney reabsorption.

increased

Absorption of calcium from the GI tract is (increased, decreased) by vitamin D.

calcium

490. Vitamin D mobilizes _____ ions from the bones.

491. In addition to vitamin D, parathyroid hormone is important in controlling the serum concentration of calcium. The parathyroid releases parathyroid hormone when there is a low serum calcium concentration. The release of the hormone subsequently draws calcium from the bones and assists with its transfer into the plasma.

suppress

Because of the feedback mechanism, a high serum calcium concentration would (stimulate, suppress) parathyroid secretion.

492. One of the functions of parathyroid hormone is to stimulate calcium and phosphate resorption from bone. This would increase serum calcium concentration.

Parathyroid hormone (stimulates, suppresses) resorp-   stimulates
tion of calcium and phosphate from bone.

493. Parathyroid hormone stimulates resorption of bone,
which involves breaking down bone to release calcium
and phosphate. Parathyroid hormone also influences the
serum calcium concentration through its effect on the kidney to increase the excretion of phosphate ions.

Parathyroid hormone (increases, decreases) the renal   increases
excretion of phosphate ions.

494. Parathyroid hormone reduces the amount of phosphate
ions that are resorbed by the kidney tubules. Therefore
more phosphate is excreted in the urine, and the serum
phosphate concentration falls.
a. Parathyroid hormone influences the kidney tubules to
   resorb (more, less) phosphate ions.   less
b. When more phosphate is excreted, the serum phos-
   phate concentration (falls, rises).   falls

495. Generally speaking, phosphate and calcium levels are re-
versed. Therefore a decrease in phosphate results in an increase in serum calcium.

Serum calcium levels increase as phosphate levels

_____.   decrease

496. So far we have considered the effect of vitamin D and of
parathyroid hormone on serum calcium levels. Let us
consider the hormone calcitonin. This hormone is secreted by the thyroid gland and reduces the blood calcium
concentration by inhibited calcium mobilization from
bone and tends to lower serum calcium levels in a way
that is opposite that of parathyroid hormone. Calcitonin
secretion is stimulated directly by a high serum calcium
level. Calcitonin is generally thought to have a weak effect on extracellular calcium.
a. The effect of calcitonin is to (increase, decrease)   decrease
   serum calcium levels.
b. The effect of parathyroid hormone is to (increase, de-   increase
   crease) serum calcium levels.
c. Therefore the effect of calcitonin and of parathyroid
   hormone on the serum calcium level is (the same,
   opposite).   opposite

CALCIUM DEFICIT (HYPOCALCEMIA)

497. A serum calcium deficit is called **hypocalcemia**. In hypocalcemia the serum calcium is below 8.5 mg/dl or at the ionized calcium level of below 4.5 mEq/L (see Table 4-2) (Figure 4-8).

10.5   a. Normal serum calcium is 8.5 to ___ mg/dl.

5.3   b. Normal ionized serum calcium is 4.5 to ___ mEq/L.

4.5   c. In hypocalcemia, the serum calcium is below ___ mEq/L.

Causes

498. A serum calcium deficit can occur from inadequate intake or from increased excretion of calcium from the body. People with pancreatic disease, alcoholism, or disease of the small intestine may fail to absorb calcium and will then excrete large amounts of calcium in the feces.

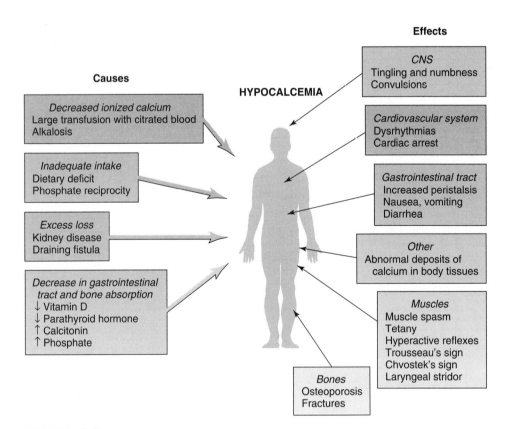

FIGURE **4-8**

Causes and effects of hypocalcemia. From Beare PG, Myers JL: *Adult health nursing*, ed 3, St Louis, 1998, Mosby.

a. Serum calcium deficit can occur from inadequate
   _____.   intake

b. Decreased absorption of calcium from the intestine
   may result in (hypo-, hyper-) calcemia.   hypo-

499. Parathyroid hormone deficiency (hypoparathyroidism),
     caused by thyroid or parathyroid surgery and/or a vita-
     min-D deficiency that results in calcium stores becoming
     depleted, and menopause, which results in a lack of estro-
     gen stimulation that leads to reabsorption of calcium into
     the bone, are potential causes of hypocalcemia.
     a. Hypocalcemia may be caused by (an excess, a deficit)   a deficit
        of parathyroid hormone.
     b. Vitamin D deficiency may result in (hypo-, hyper-)   hypo-
        calcemia.
     c. Menopause (can, cannot) cause a calcium deficit.   can

500. Phosphates administered either intravenously or rec-
     tally/orally will result in hypocalcemia as phosphate
     binds with calcium.
         Giving phosphate intravenously will result in
         _____.   hypocalcemia

501. We have looked at inadequate intake, decreased absorp-
     tion, pancreatic disease, disease of the small intestine,
     parathyroid hormone deficiency, vitamin D deficiency,
     and the infusion of phosphate given intravenously as pos-
     sible causes of hypocalcemia.
         Of the following, which may cause hypocalcemia?
     _____ a. Decreased intestinal absorption   a
     _____ b. Pancreatic disease   b
     _____ c. Hyperactive parathyroids
     _____ d. Vitamin D deficiency   d
     _____ e. Phosphate-containing intravenous fluids   e

502. Other possible causes of hypocalcemia include the use of
     loop diuretics that promote renal excretion of calcium; the
     medication calcitonin, which decreases the resorption of
     calcium from the bone; and the administration of a blood
     transfusion that has had citrate added to it (to prevent clot-
     ting), which binds with calcium making it unavailable for
     use elsewhere in the body.
         Hypocalcemia may be caused by _____,   loop diuretics
         _____, and _____.   calcitonin
                                                                 citrate

503. Other causes of hypocalcemia are alkalosis, which may
     cause calcium to bind to albumin, and renal insufficiency,

hypo-

which may lead to a decrease in the ability to activate vitamin D and the inability to excrete phosphorus (normally leading to hyperphosphatemia). When hyperphosphatemia occurs, (hyper-, hypo-) calcemia follows.

REMEMBER: When the phosphorus level rises, the serum calcium level falls.

Edetate disodium
burns
draining intestinal
fistulas

504. Finally hypocalcemia can result from the treatment of lead poisoning with administration of edetate disodium, which binds with calcium as it is excreted; from burns because calcium is being held in the ECF space and therefore is not present in the serum; and from draining intestinal fistulas.

_____, _____ and _____
may lead to hypocalcemia.

Signs and Symptoms

tetany

505. The signs and symptoms of hypocalcemia include those associated with neural excitability, such as muscle spasms and tingling sensations. As the deficit increases, significant skeletal, cardiac, and smooth muscle excitability may have a serious effect on homeostasis. Tetany is considered the most characteristic sign of hypocalcemia.
    A characteristic sign of hypocalcemia is _____.

cramps
hyper-

506. The signs and symptoms of increased excitability include paresthesias, especially numbness or tingling of the feet and hands; skeletal muscle cramps; abdominal spasms and cramps; hyperactive reflexes; and convulsions (Figure 4-9).
    a. Neural excitability that occurs in hypocalcemia may be evidenced by muscle and abdominal _____.
    b. Reflexes will be (hyper-, hypo-) active.

hypo-
carpal spasm

507. Trousseau's sign may be present in persons with hypocalcemia. To test for Trousseau's sign, a blood pressure cuff is applied to the upper arm and the cuff is inflated above the systolic level for 3 minutes. A positive sign is the development of carpal spasm (Figure 4-10). The person's thumb adducts, and the fingers contract.
    a. Trousseau's sign may be present in persons with (hypo-, hyper-) calcemia.
    b. A positive Trousseau's sign is demonstrated by _____
    _____.

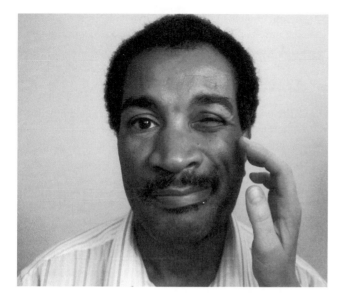

FIGURE 4-9
Facial muscle response—positive Chvostek's sign in hypocalcemia. From Ignatavicius D, Workman M, Mishler M: *Medical-surgical nursing across the health care continuum*, ed 3, Philadelphia, 1999, WB Saunders.

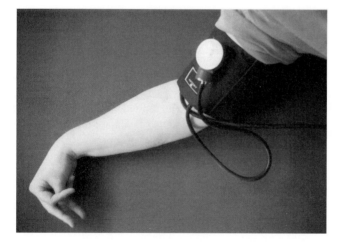

FIGURE 4-10
Palmar flexion—positive Trousseau's sign in hypocalcemia. From Ignatavicius D, Workman M, Mishler M: *Medical-surgical nursing across the health care continuum*, ed 3, Philadelphia, 1999, WB Saunders.

508. Chvostek's sign also may be used to observe an increase in neuromuscular excitability (see Figure 4-9).

A positive Chvostek's sign indicates (an increase, a decrease) in neuromuscular excitability.   an increase

REMEMBER: Chvostek's sign is elicited by tapping just in front of the ear over the facial nerve. A positive sign occurs when a spasm of the lip, nose, and eyelid occurs.

509. Mental changes occurring in hypocalcemia may include changes in mood, emotional depression, impairment of memory, confusion, or hallucinations.

hypo-

Emotional depression or confusion may be evidenced in (hypo-, hyper-) calcemia.

510. If the calcium deficit is prolonged, then calcium will be withdrawn from the bones to increase the extracellular calcium. In a prolonged calcium deficit, calcium will be

the bones   mobilized from _____.

511. Osteoporosis (loss of bone density) may result in a decrease in skeletal height and an increase in the potential for pathologic fractures. Additionally, a prolonged lack of calcium may lead to structural change in skeletal mass and may be related to a sedentary lifestyle, lack of exercise, low calcium intake, vitamin D deficiency, and excessive fat intake.

increased   a. When osteoporosis is present, the potential for pathologic fractures is (increased, decreased).

may   b. The loss of skeletal mass (may, may not) be related to the individual's lifestyle.

512. During adolescence and after the age of 40 there is a need for an increase in calcium intake. For the adolescent the need is related to the increase in maximum bone mass and calcium deposit, and, for an individual over 40, especially a woman, increased amounts of calcium are used to supplement calcium resorption that occurs.

What two age groups in particular need to supplement their calcium intake?

adolescents   a. _____

those over 40   b. _____

513. In hypocalcemia there is a decrease in cardiac output and an abnormal electrocardiographic finding such as a prolonged S-T interval.

a. An electrocardiographic finding that is characteristic

S-T   of hypocalcemia is a prolonged ____ interval.

decrease   b. There is a _____ in cardiac output in hypocalcemia.

514. It is important to observe for hypocalcemia in patients who have had recent surgery involving the parathyroid or thyroid glands or removal of the parathyroid glands and in patients who have sustained injury to these glands as a result of trauma or radiation treatments. The serum calcium level after injury or remov-

al of the glands may drop rapidly and result in convulsions.

After surgery involving the thyroid or parathyroid
glands, patients should be observed for signs and symptoms of (hypo-, hyper-) calcemia.

hypo-

515. Patients who are undergoing hemodialysis, which may
cause them to excrete more urine and calcium, and who
may receive blood that is preserved with citrate should be
observed for signs and symptoms of hypocalcemia. Additionally, individuals who are taking anticonvulsants such
as Dilantin and phenobarbital are at risk for hypocalcemia
because these medications may hinder calcium absorption and vitamin D metabolism.

Hypocalcemia may develop in patients who are undergoing _____ or who are taking medications such
as _____ or _____ .

hemodialysis
Dilantin
phenobarbital

Treatment

516. Acute hypocalcemia is usually treated by correcting the
imbalance and identifying the underlying cause. Immediate treatment is begun with calcium gluconate or calcium
chloride, given intravenously. When administering IV calcium replacement, it is important that the nurse clarify first
which replacement, calcium gluconate or calcium chloride, is to be given IV; calcium chloride contains three
times the amount of available calcium as calcium gluconate. The IV calcium replacement should be placed in a
solution of 5% dextrose only. Normal saline will increase
calcium loss, and a solution that has bicarbonate in it will
precipitate. The solution should be administered slowly according to the physician's orders; rapid infusion may be fatal. While administering calcium intravenously, the nurse
should watch for signs and symptoms of hypercalcemia.

a. _____ and _____ are the intravenous drugs of choice for hypocalcemia.

Calcium gluconate
calcium chloride

b. Either calcium gluconate or calcium chloride (should,
should not) be diluted in dextrose 5%.

should

c. While administering IV calcium replacement, the
nurse should observe the patient for (hypo-, or hyper-)
calcemia.

hyper-

517. Treatment of chronic hypocalcemia will include oral calcium supplements to increase the calcium level or vitamin
D supplements to promote the GI absorption of calcium.

Calcium supplements (may, may not) be given orally
in treatment of chronic hypocalcemia.

may

518. In patients who are digitalized, calcium salts should be given cautiously, and the patient must be observed continuously on a cardiac monitor. Calcium has an effect on the heart similar to that of digitalis. The arrhythmias that may occur include premature atrial or ventricular contractions, sinus bradycardia, and ventricular tachycardia.

a. Calcium has an effect on the heart similar to that of

digitalis _____.

b. A digitalized patient must be observed on a cardiac

calcium monitor, especially when _____ supplements are given intravenously.

CONCEPT CHECK

Although calcium is the most abundant cation in the body, 99% of that calcium is in the bones. The 1% of calcium in the blood remains remarkably constant. The ionized calcium is needed to help maintain the permeability of cell membranes for the transmission of nerve impulses and neuromuscular excitability and for normal cardiac function. Also, calcium is necessary for blood coagulation, activating enzyme reactions, and hormone secretion.

Normally calcium is ingested with the diet and absorbed through the GI tract. Serum calcium is gained by resorption of bone and by renal tubular resorption. Serum calcium is lost by renal and GI excretion and by bone deposition. Major factors that control serum calcium concentration are vitamin D, parathyroid hormone, calcitonin, and serum concentrations of calcium and phosphate ions.

A serum calcium deficit can occur as a result of inadequate intake or from decreased absorption. Hypocalcemia may result from a deficiency of parathyroid hormone or of vitamin D. The signs and symptoms of hypocalcemia include those associated with neural excitability. Tetany is the most characteristic sign of hypocalcemia; therefore nursing care must include careful observation of the patient to detect increasing neuromuscular excitability. Hypocalcemia is usually treated with a calcium salt such as calcium gluconate.

INFORMATION CHECK

calcium   1. The most abundant cation in the body is _____.

essential   2. Calcium is (essential, not essential) for the transmission of nerve impulses.

tetany   3. The most characteristic sign of hypocalcemia is _____.

4. In caring for a patient with a potential for hypocalcemia, an
   important nursing action is _____.   observation

Calcium Excess (Hypercalcemia)

519. **Hypercalcemia** exists whenever the ionized calcium is
     over 5.0 mEq/L or serum calcium is over 10.5 mg/dl.
     a. Hypercalcemia is indicated by an ionized calcium
        level above ___ mEq/L.   5.0
     b. A serum calcium level over ___ mg/dl indicates   10.5
        hypercalcemia.

Causes

520. There are two significant causes of hypercalcemia: (1) hy-
     perparathyroidism, which increases calcium resorption
     from the bone, calcium reabsorption from the kidneys,
     and calcium absorption from the intestines, and (2) neo-
     plastic diseases, in which malignant cells invading the
     bones release a parathyroid-like hormone that causes an
     increase in serum calcium levels.

     _____ and _____ are two   Hyperparathyroidism
     significant causes of hypercalcemia.   neoplastic disease

521. Although metastasis of cancer cells to bone may cause the
     breakdown of bone and the release of excessive calcium,
     cancer also may cause hypercalcemia without bone
     metastasis. Many malignant tumors produce inappropri-
     ate hormones. Some tumors produce a parathyroid-like
     substance that causes increased bone resorption and a rise
     in the serum calcium concentration.

     Causes of excessive release of calcium from bone are:
     a. Cancer with _____ to bone   metastasis
     b. Production of a _____-like hormone from the   parathyroid
        tumor

522. Bone destruction may exceed bone production to the ex-
     tent that the kidneys are unable to excrete the excessive
     calcium ions. Also, hypercalcemia may result from a pri-
     mary hyperparathyroidism, which may be caused by a be-
     nign adenoma of one or more parathyroid glands.
     a. Primary hyperparathyroidism may be caused by a
        _____ adenoma.   benign
     b. Hyperparathyroidism will result in (hypo-, hyper-)   hyper-
        calcemia.

523. Hypercalcemia also can result from excessive intake of
     calcium or vitamin D or because of a condition such as

hyperthyroidism, that promotes the release of calcium from bone into the ECF.

excessive

a. Hypercalcemia can result from (excessive, inadequate) intake of calcium.

b. Excessive vitamin D intake can result in (hypo-,

hyper-

hyper-) calcemia.

c. Conditions that promote the release of calcium from

hypercalcemia

bones can result in _____.

Hyperthyroidism

d. _____ can lead to hypercalcemia.

524. Excessive calcium intake may occur in patients with peptic ulcer disease treated with milk and alkaline antacids, especially calcium carbonate, for long periods and in individuals who have been taking lithium or thiazide diuretics, which decrease the excretion of calcium from the kidneys.

a. A person with peptic ulcer disease who is treated with milk and calcium carbonate may develop (hyper-,

hypo-

hypo-) calcemia.

Lithium

b. _____ and _____ decrease the excretion of

thiazide diuretics

calcium from the kidneys.

525. Another cause of hypercalcemia is prolonged immobilization. Remember, we learned that bone deposition or formation occurs in response to stress and strain. Therefore with disuse there is increased bone resorption and also decreased bone formation.

hyper-

a. Prolonged immobilization may result in (hyper-, hypo-) calcemia.

increased

b. Disuse causes (increased, decreased) bone resorption.

decreased

c. Disuse results in (increased, decreased) bone formation.

526. In considering the causes of hypercalcemia, we have looked at factors related to excessive intake of calcium, increased bone destruction, and decreased bone formation. Other causes of hypercalcemia are the use of diuretics, endocrine disorders, and renal diseases.

Some factors that lead to hypercalcemia are:

a

_____ a. Excessive intake of calcium

_____ b. Decreased bone destruction

c

_____ c. Decreased bone formation

d

_____ d. Use of diuretics

e

_____ e. Renal diseases

Signs and Symptoms

527. The signs and symptoms of hypercalcemia result from three sources: a decrease in neuromuscular activity, re-

sorption of calcium from bone, and the effect of high calcium concentrations on the kidney. Symptoms are usually
more extreme if the level is greater than 15 mg/dl or if the
symptoms developed acutely.

The three sources of signs and symptoms of hypercalcemia are:

a. (A decrease, An increase) in neuromuscular activity   A decrease
b. (Resorption, Deposition) of calcium from (in) bone   Resorption
c. Effect of (high, low) calcium concentration on the   high
   kidney
d. Signs and symptoms are usually (more, less) extreme   more
   when the serum calcium level is 15 mg/dl or when the
   signs and symptoms begin suddenly.

528. The decreased neuromuscular activity will be evidenced
     in generalized skeletal and cardiac muscle and nervous
     system weakness, lethargy, loss of muscle tone, and
     ataxia. The person may show mental confusion, impair-
     ment of memory, slurred speech, personality or behavior
     changes, stupor, or coma (Figure 4-11).
     a. In hypercalcemia generalized muscle weakness results
        from the (increased, decreased) neuromuscular activity.   decreased
     b. Stupor or coma may result from (hypo-, hyper-)   hyper-
        calcemia.

529. The heart responds to hypercalcemia with effects like
     those of digitalis use. Bradycardia and increased contrac-
     tility occur in hypercalcemia. On the electrocardiogram,
     the Q-T interval shortens and the T waves invert. Ventric-
     ular arrhythmias may develop.
     a. Cardiac effects of hypercalcemia may include (brady-,   brady-
        tachy-) cardia.
     b. The Q-T interval on the electrocardiogram (lengthens,
        shortens).   shortens
     c. With hypercalcemia, ventricular _____ may   arrhythmias
        develop.

530. The GI symptoms of hypercalcemia include anorexia,
     nausea, vomiting, and constipation. The patient exhibits a
     decrease in bowel sounds and may develop a paralytic
     ileus.

     Hypercalcemia may have symptoms including anorex-
     ia, nausea, vomiting, and (constipation, diarrhea).   constipation

531. The signs and symptoms related to resorption of cal-
     cium from bone include deep bone pain, radiographic ev-

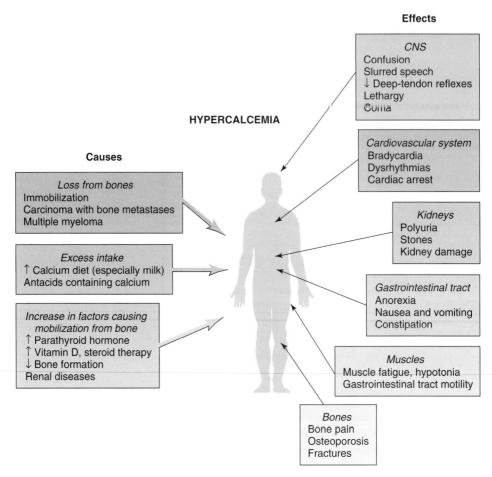

FIGURE 4-11
Causes and effects of hypercalcemia. From Beare PG, Myers JL: *Adult health nursing*, ed 3, St Louis, 1998, Mosby.

idence of bone demineralization, and potentially pathologic fractures.

Deep bone pain may be caused by resorption of _____ from the bone.

calcium

532. High extracellular concentrations of calcium impair the ability of the kidney to concentrate urine. The polyuria that results from hypercalcemia will lead to the need for increased intake of water.

a. When the kidney is less able to concentrate urine, (polyuria, anuria) will be evident.

polyuria

b. Polyuria (will, will not) lead to the need for increased water intake.

will

533. Hypercalcemia predisposes patients to the development of renal calculi (kidney stones) and other calcifications.
    Renal calculi may be the result of (hyper-, hypo-) calcemia.

hyper-

> **REMEMBER:** A significant increase in calcium is potentially fatal.

Hypercalcemic crisis is an emergency condition caused by an acute increase in serum calcium levels above 8 to 9 mEq/L; signs and symptoms of this emergency condition include intractable nausea, dehydration, stupor, and coma. Azotemia is present and hypokalemia and/or hypomagnesemia also may be present along with hypernatremia because of water loss.
    a. Hypercalcemic crisis may occur if the serum calcium rises above _ to _ mEq/L.

8, 9

    b. Intractable nausea and vomiting will lead to a (deficit, excess) in fluid volume.

deficit

    c. Another electrolyte imbalance likely to be present is (hypo-, hyper-) kalemia.

hypo-

535. In patients with hypercalcemic crisis, mortality has been high. Death often results from cardiac arrest.
    Mortality is (high, low) in patients with hypercalcemic crisis.

high

Treatment

536. Treating hypercalcemia involves removing the cause or controlling the condition that caused the excess serum calcium. When hypercalcemia is severe, the first thing to receive attention is the need for hydration. This will reduce the risk of renal damage and may reduce the serum calcium by dilution. Hemodialysis or peritoneal dialysis that is calcium-free or has only a small amount of calcium may be necessary to remove the increased calcium.
    When hypercalcemia is severe, _____ must be adequate to reduce the possible renal damage.

hydration

537. Normal saline given intravenously will provide hydration as well as produce some urinary excretion of calcium because the kidneys selectively resorb sodium.
    The intravenous solution used to provide hydration in hypercalcemia is _____.

normal saline

538. When normal saline is given intravenously, it is important to match the rate and amount of saline solution to the patient's urine output. You need to measure the patient's hourly, as well as total, urine output.

hourly

When normal saline is given intravenously to treat hypercalcemia, you should measure the urine output _____ (frequency).

539. If normal saline does not produce adequate diuresis, then diuretics such as furosemide (Lasix) may be given to increase the excretion of calcium.

furosemide (Lasix)

Diuretics such as _____ may be used to increase the excretion of calcium.

540. Phosphate also is used to lower the serum calcium level. Phosphate promotes deposition of calcium in bone and decreases intestinal absorption. However, a side effect of oral phosphate ingestion is diarrhea. Intravenous infusions of phosphate are used only for hypercalcemic crisis because of potential for soft tissue calcification and renal failure if the serum calcium decreases acutely.

a. The substance that acts by promoting deposition of calcium in bone and decreases intestinal absorption is

phosphate

_____.

b. Intravenous infusions of phosphate are used only for

hypercalcemic

_____ crisis.

541. Corticosteroids (Cortef) and mithramycin (Mithracin) are used for treating hypercalcemia in persons with cancer. Mithramycin is a potent antitumor drug that shares the cytotoxicities of other antitumor drugs but does lower serum calcium concentration. Corticosteroids and mithramycin are used for treating hypercalcemia in persons with

cancer

_____.

542. In giving care to a person with hypercalcemia, it is important to protect him or her from pathologic fractures. Positioning and moving must be done with extreme care to prevent fractures.

A potential problem for persons with hypercalcemia is

fractures

pathologic _____.

543. Formation of calcium stones in the urinary tract is another potential problem for persons with hypercalcemia. Persons with hypercalcemia should be encouraged to drink

3000 to 4000 ml of water per day to reduce the possibility of renal calculi.

a. Persons with hypercalcemia may develop _____ in the urinary tract.

calculi

b. Persons with hypercalcemia should drink ____ to ____ ml of water per day.

3000, 4000

544. Acidic urine will help to decrease the possibility of urinary stone formation. Foods such as prunes or cranberry juice or ascorbic acid will favor increased acidity in the urine.

a. Urinary stone formation is more likely in (acidic, alkaline) urine.

alkaline

b. Persons with hypercalcemia should eat foods that will help produce (acidic, alkaline) urine.

acidic

545. Urinary tract infections should be avoided. Good perineal care and meticulous catheter care are especially important for persons with hypercalcemia.

Good perineal care and meticulous catheter care will help prevent urinary tract _____.

infections

✓ CONCEPT CHECK

Hypercalcemia can be the result of excessive calcium intake, excessive vitamin D intake, or conditions that promote release of calcium from the bones. Whenever bone destruction exceeds bone production to the extent that the kidneys are unable to excrete the excess calcium ions, hypercalcemia may result.

The signs and symptoms of hypercalcemia result from a decrease in neuromuscular activity, resorption of calcium from bone, and the effect on the kidney of high serum calcium concentrations. Decreased neuromuscular activity may be evidenced by generalized muscle weakness, loss of muscle tone, mental confusion, and coma. The cardiac signs of hypercalcemia include bradycardia, increased contractility, and ventricular arrhythmias. The increased resorption of bone is evidenced by deep bone pain and radiographic evidence of bone demineralization. The effect on the kidney is indicated by decreased concentration of urine, increased urine output, and renal calculi.

Hypercalcemic crisis is caused by a rapid increase in serum calcium levels. Adequate hydration must be provided. Diuretics and/or phosphate may be used to treat hypercalcemic crisis.

In caring for patients with hypercalcemia, it is important to protect them from pathologic fractures. Urinary tract infections should be prevented. Intake of water should be in the amount of 3000 to 4000 ml/day.

INFORMATION CHECK

1. Three causes of hypercalcemia are:

excessive intake of calcium

a. _____

excessive intake of vitamin D

b. _____

release of calcium from bone

c. _____

2. The signs and symptoms of hypercalcemia include (a decrease, an increase) in neuromuscular activity.

a decrease

3. The increased resorption of bone is evidenced by:

deep bone pain

a. _____

radiographic evidence of demineralization

b. _____

4. Patients with hypercalcemia should be moved gently because of the potential for _____.

pathologic fractures

5. A patient with hypercalcemia should have a daily fluid intake of _____ to _____ ml.

3000, 4000

PHOSPHORUS IMBALANCE

546. Phosphorus is the primary anion in the intracellular fluid. Approximately 85% of phosphorus in the body is combined with calcium in the bones and teeth and 14% is in soft tissues. Less than 1% of the body's phosphorus is in the ECF.

    The amount of phosphorus that is in the serum is less than _%.

1

547. Although the amount of phosphorus in the ECF is small, the portion inside cells is large. Phosphorus supports several metabolic functions, including maintenance of acid-base balance by way of the phosphate buffer system. It functions in the formation of energy-storing substances, such as creatine phosphate and adenosine triphosphate (ATP). Phosphorus is needed in the formation of red blood cells (RBCs) and acts as an intermediary in the metabolism of carbohydrates, proteins, and fats. It is essential to normal nerve and muscle function and to cell membrane integrity. Phosphorus is essential for red blood cell delivery of oxygen to the body, structural support for bones and teeth, white blood cell phagocytosis, and platelet function.

Phosphorus is (essential, not essential) to many func-   essential
tions within the body.

548. Nearly all phosphorus in the body is in the form of phos-
     phate (PO_4); the terms phosphorus and phosphate are
     used interchangeably. Serum phosphate levels may vary
     with gender, age, and diet. These levels decrease with age,
     except for a slight rise in women after menopause. When
     glucose and insulin are introduced into the plasma, serum
     phosphate shifts into cells, temporarily decreasing its
     concentration in the ECF. Acid-base imbalances affect
     serum phosphorus levels. For example, respiratory alka-
     losis causes a shift of phosphorus into cells that may re-
     sult in hypophosphatemia.
     a. The terms phosphorus and phosphate (are, are not)   are
        used interchangeably.
     b. Shifts of phosphorus from plasma into cells may result
        in (hyper-, hypo-) phosphatemia.   hypo-

549. The level of serum phosphate is influenced by dietary in-
     take, intestinal absorption, hormonally regulated bone re-
     sorption and deposition, and renal excretion. Approxi-
     mately 90% of the phosphorus that is excreted is in the
     urine, whereas the other 10% is excreted in the feces. The
     normal range of serum phosphorus is 2.5 to 4.5 mg/dl.
     a. The majority of phosphorus is excreted from the

        _____.   kidneys
     b. The normal range of serum phosphorus is ___ to ___   2.5, 4.5
        mg/dl.

        Additionally the amount of phosphorus ingested is
     generally the same as the amount absorbed, and the
     parathyroid hormone, in response to altered calcium, af-
     fects phosphorus with its regulation of calcium because
     the two have an opposing relationship.

PHOSPHORUS DEFICIT (HYPOPHOSPHATEMIA)

550. In **hypophosphatemia**, the serum phosphorus will be less
     than 2.5 mg/dl.
     a. Normal serum phosphorus levels are ___ to ___ mg/dl.   2.5, 4.5
     b. In hypophosphatemia the serum phosphorus levels are
        less than ___ mg/dl.   2.5

Causes
551. A serum deficit of phosphorus, called hypophospha-
     temia, may be caused by increased renal excretion of

phosphate, a shift of phosphorus from the extracellular to the intracellular space, or by a decrease in intestinal absorption. Hyperparathyroidism and renal failure and thiazide and loop diuretics cause an increased loss of phosphorus in the urine. Some specific causes of hypophosphatemia are intestinal malabsorption, which may be associated with vitamin D deficiency, use of magnesium- and aluminum-containing antacids that bind phosphorus, chronic alcohol abuse, or malabsorption syndromes; diabetic ketoacidosis, resulting in loss of phosphorus through the kidneys in response to high glucose levels; and respiratory alkalosis, causing the use of phosphorus by cells to be accelerated when glucose is metabolized.

Which of the following may cause hypophosphatemia?

a   _____ a. Malabsorption syndromes
     _____ b. Increased renal resorption of phosphate
c   _____ c. Respiratory alkalosis
d   _____ d. Vitamin-D deficiency
     _____ e. Hypoparathyroidism
f   _____ f. Thiazide and loop diuretic use
g   _____ g. Diabetic ketoacidosis

552. Subsequently, a phosphate deficiency may cause serum magnesium to be decreased because of increased urinary excretion of magnesium and may therefore produce skeletal changes such as rickets or osteomalacia that may be evident on x-ray films.

may   A decrease in serum phosphate (may, may not) be linked with skeletal changes.

Signs and Symptoms

553. The signs and symptoms of hypophosphatemia may occur quickly or slowly and generally appear in many systems. For the most part hypophosphatemia results in musculoskeletal, CNS, hematologic, and cardiac alterations. They are related to a deficiency of ATP and a low energy source and the enzyme 2,3-diphosphoglycerate (2,3-DPG). As an enzyme in the RBCs, 2,3-DPG interacts with hemoglobin to promote oxygen release, and a deficiency of this enzyme impairs oxygen delivery to the body tissues, whereas a lack of ATP results in an impairment of cellular energy resources. CNS and muscular changes related to hypophosphatemia include muscle weakness, tremors, paresthesias, confusion, and seizures.

Which of the following are signs and symptoms of hypophosphatemia?

_____ a. Muscle weakness   a

_____ b. Confusion   b

_____ c. Tetany

554. The central nervous system and muscles are affected by hypophosphatemia. There are also hematologic abnormalities that include tissue hypoxia, hemolytic anemia related to the structure of the RBC, possible infection as a result of low ATP in the white blood cells, and possible bleeding, especially GI bleeding, caused by poor platelet function. Cardiopulmonary effects include cardiomyopathies and respiratory failure as the cardiac and respiratory muscles become weakened. Signs of chronic hypophosphatemia also include memory loss caused by the lack of ATP to the CNS and bone pain resulting from the loss of bone density.

   a. Hypophosphatemia impairs oxygen delivery to tissues, which may be evidenced in tissue (oxygenation, hypoxia).   hypoxia

   b. Signs of chronic hypophosphatemia may include

       _____ and _____.   memory loss
                                                               bone pain

Treatment

555. Treatment of hypophosphatemia involves identifying and treating the cause and correcting the imbalance. If a person has had an inadequate intake of phosphorus, foods high in phosphorus might be given. These foods include meats, fish, milk and milk products, whole grains, nuts, and dried beans.

   Which of the following foods are high in phosphorus?

_____ a. Fruits

_____ b. Meats   b

_____ c. Milk   c

_____ d. Carrots

_____ e. Whole grains   e

556. Foods high in phosphorus may be used in some situations but oral phosphate supplements such as Netra-Phos may also be given. A person with low phosphorus should avoid phosphate-binding antacids because they interfere with intestinal absorption of phosphorus. Intravenous sodium phosphate or potassium phosphate may be needed in cases of severe hypophosphatemia. Concentrated intravenous phosphates are hypertonic and must be diluted.

Potassium phosphate is given at a rate of no more than 10 mEq/hr. The dosage is generally based on the patient's serum phosphorus. It is important to realize that many precautions are necessary when giving phosphate intravenously. It is contraindicated for persons with hypocalcemia and hyperphosphatemia.

diluted

a. Intravenous phosphates are hypertonic and must be _____.

hypernatremia

b. Intravenous phosphates are contraindicated in hypocalcemia and _____.

557. It is important for the nurse to assess the patient at risk for developing hypophosphatemia. Assess for signs and symptoms of hypoxia, such as restlessness, confusion, and chest pain. Monitor the patient's respiratory rate and depth. Report significant changes.

are

Careful monitoring and safety measures (are, are not) indicated for a patient who either has hypophosphatemia or is at risk for developing it.

✓Concept Check

The primary anion in the intracellular fluid is phosphorus. Less than 1% of the total body phosphorus is in the intravascular fluids. Phosphorus is essential to many functions within the body, including acid-base balance, formation of ATP and RBCs, metabolism of nutrients, normal nerve and muscle function, and structural support for bones and teeth.

Hypophosphatemia may be caused by renal failure or hyperparathyroidism. Decreased intestinal absorption associated with vitamin D deficiency, increased urinary excretion, or increased phosphorus use may cause a deficit of phosphorus.

Normal serum phosphorus levels are 2.5 to 4.5 mg/dl. In hypophosphatemia the serum levels will be below 2.5 mg/dl. Because phosphorus is essential to many functions in the body, the signs and symptoms of hypophosphatemia may include impaired cellular energy resources, tissue hypoxia, hemolytic anemia, possible infection, and possible bleeding. Cardiopulmonary effects include cardiomyopathies and respiratory failure. Muscle weakness, tremors, paresthesias, confusion, and seizures may occur. Memory loss and bone pain may occur in chronic hypophosphatemia.

Treatment of hypophosphatemia includes identifying and treating the cause as well as providing sources of phosphates.

Nursing care involves assessing for signs of hypoxia, cardiopulmonary changes, and muscle and neurologic changes as well as providing care to prevent injury.

✓ *INFORMATION CHECK*

1. The amount of the total body phosphorus that is in the serum is less than __%.   1

2. The normal range of serum phosphorus is ___ to ___ mg/dl.   1.7, 2.6

3. Which of the following require normal phosphorus levels in order to function correctly?
   _____ a. Acid-base balance   a
   _____ b. Formation of ATP   b
             c. Metabolism of nutrients   c
   _____ d. Normal nerve and muscle function   d
   _____ e. Formation of RBCs   e

4. Hypophosphatemia impairs oxygen delivery to tissues, which is evident in tissue _____.   hypoxia

5. A person with hypophosphatemia is at high risk for injury related to confusion, muscle weakness, and _____.   seizure

PHOSPHORUS EXCESS (HYPERPHOSPHATEMIA)

558. An excess of phosphorus, called **hyperphosphatemia**, greater than 4.5 mg/dl most often occurs when renal insufficiency exists and the kidneys are unable to excrete excess phosphorus. Either acute or chronic renal failure may be responsible for hyperphosphatemia.
    Hyperphosphatemia is often caused by ___ failure.   renal

Causes
559. Along with renal failure, a high phosphorus intake, which may occur via intravenous administration may result in hyperphosphatemia. When enemas containing sodium phosphate are given, increased absorption of phosphate may occur through the large intestine. Because phosphorus leaks from RBCs during storage, blood transfusions may increase the extracellular phosphorus. Large vitamin D intake leads to hyperphosphatemia because it increases the absorption of phosphorus.
    Renal failure is the most common cause of hyper

phosphatemia, but it also can be caused by which of the following?

a

     _____ a. High intake of phosphorus

     _____ b. Decreased dietary intake of phosphorus

c

     _____ c. Enemas containing sodium phosphate

d

     _____ d. Blood transfusions

     _____ e. Deficiency of vitamin D

560. An additional cause of hyperphosphatemia is injury to muscle tissue, which causes necrosis and the release of phosphorus into the ECF. Intracellular phosphates also may be released as a result of chemotherapy, which causes cell destruction. Certain endocrine disorders can cause hyperphosphatemia, such as hypoparathyroidism in which there is a decrease in the production and release of parathyroid hormone that leads to serum calcium deficiency and hence an increase in phosphate concentration because the kidneys are not excreting phosphorus. When phosphates are given intravenously or by enema administration, hyperphosphatemia results in hypocalcemia.

       An injury to muscle tissue causing necrosis may cause hyperphosphatemia because phosphorus is released from

cells   ____.

hyper- 561. When hypocalcemia exists, (hypo-, hyper-) phosphatemia is likely to occur.

562. When severe hyperphosphatemia exists, serum phosphate levels will be greater than 6.0 mg/dl. Hypocalcemia that may develop if the hyperphosphatemia is severe and occurs suddenly can produce a significant health risk.

6.0   If the level is greater than ___mg/dl, the hyperphosphatemia is considered significant.

Signs and Symptoms

563. The signs and symptoms of hyperphosphatemia are usually those seen with hypocalcemia. Anorexia, nausea, and vomiting, as well as muscle weakness and signs of neural excitability, may occur.

       The signs and symptoms of hyperphosphatemia are the

hypo- same as those in (hypo-, hyper-) calcemia.

564. When an individual has chronic hyperphosphatemia, phosphorus binds with calcium to form deposits of calcium phosphate. These deposits may occur in the heart, lungs, soft tissues, joints, and arteries. Signs of these cal-

cifications include corneal haziness, conjunctivitis, irregular heart rate, and oliguria.

Corneal haziness, conjunctivitis, irregular heart rate, and oliguria may be found in persons with hyperphosphatemia and are caused by deposits of _____ _____ in the soft tissues.

calcium phosphate

Treatment

565. The treatment of hyperphosphatemia is directed at the underlying disorder when possible. Foods that are high in phosphorus should be avoided. In severe cases, intravenous administration of calcium along with the use of dialysis to remove excess phosphorus may be necessary. Aluminum hydroxide gels bind with phosphorus in the intestine and may sometimes be used in persons in renal failure.

REMEMBER: An elevated phosphate level in a patient with chronic renal failure may help increase the oxygenation of the patient by allowing more oxygen to move from the RBCs to the tissues.

In hyperphosphatemia, the treatment is aimed at limiting the intake of phosphorus, binding phosphorus present, and/or removing excess phosphorus through the use of _____.

dialysis

566. Nursing care includes monitoring the serum phosphate and calcium levels in patients at risk for calcium phosphate calcifications. Note abnormal values, assess for signs and symptoms of hyperphosphatemia, and report to the physician. Measure urine output regularly, because hyperphosphatemia can impair renal function.

Nursing care includes monitoring serum phosphate and calcium levels, reporting abnormal values, assessing for signs and symptoms of hyperphosphatemia, and careful measuring of _____.

urine output

✓ CONCEPT CHECK

Hyperphosphatemia most often occurs when the kidneys are unable to excrete excess phosphorus. Other causes include high intake of phosphorus (which may occur via intravenous administration), high intake of vitamin D, and blood transfusions. Sodium phosphate given as an enema may lead to increased absorption, and injury to cells may lead to the release of intracellular phosphorus.

Because the serum calcium level falls in hyperphosphatemia, the signs and symptoms will be the same as those in hypocalcemia. In persons with long-term hyperphosphatemia, deposits of calcium phosphate may occur in soft tissues, joints, and arteries. These primarily affect the eyes, heart, and kidneys.

Treatment is aimed at limiting the intake of phosphorus, binding the phosphorus present, and/or removing excess phosphorus through the use of dialysis. Nursing care includes monitoring serum phosphate and calcium levels, reporting abnormal values, assessing for signs and symptoms of hyperphosphatemia, and measuring urine output.

INFORMATION CHECK

1. The most common cause of hyperphosphatemia is renal _____.

failure

2. When the serum level of phosphorus increases, the serum level of calcium _____.

decreases

3. In persons with long-term hyperphosphatemia, deposits of _____ may occur in soft tissues, joints, and blood vessels.

calcium phosphate

4. The serum phosphate level in hyperphosphatemia will be above ___ mg/dl.

6.0

5. In addition to assessing the patient, the nurse will regularly measure the _____.

urine output

KEY POINTS

1. Electrolytes are essential for promotion of neuromuscular function, maintenance of body fluid osmolality, regulation of acid-base balance, and distribution of body fluids and electrolytes.

2. Sodium is the main extracellular cation and is essential for transmission of impulses in nerve and muscle fibers, control of cell size, and maintenance of ECF volume.

3. Potassium is the main intracellular cation and is necessary to maintain intracellular fluid volume; regulate neuromuscular function especially the cardiac muscle; and maintain hydrogen ion concentration.

4. Magnesium is the second most abundant cation in the intracellular compartment and is an activator in enzyme reactions, especially carbohydrate metabolism. It is required for synthesis of nucleic acids and proteins, and it is important for normal neuromuscular function. Magnesium also influences levels of intracellular calcium and facilitates transport of sodium and potassium across cell membranes.

5. Calcium is found primarily in the bones; however, the small amount of extracellular calcium is needed to maintain the permeability of cell membranes for transmission of nerve impulses and neuromuscular function. Calcium aids in normal cardiac function, blood coagulation, activation of enzyme reactions, and hormone secretion.

6. Phosphorus is the primary anion in the intracellular compartment and is essential for acid-base balance, formation of ATP and RBCs, metabolism of nutrients, normal neuromuscular function, and structural support for bones and teeth.

? CRITICAL THINKING QUESTIONS

1. One of the important functions of sodium is to maintain the _____ and concentration of ECF.

volume

2. If hyponatremia is present, there may be a true deficit of sodium and/or a (loss, gain) of water.

gain

3. Mrs. Leota had a stroke that resulted in aphasia (inability to speak). When she was transferred from the hospital to a chronic care facility, her electrolytes were normal. She received tube feedings for nutrition, and no drugs were given. Mrs. Leota was readmitted to the hospital several weeks later because of hypovolemia. Her serum sodium was 156 mEq/L, and her output was 3000 to 4000 ml/day.

   a. Because of the stroke and the aphasia, Mrs. Leota was unable to indicate any sense of _____, which could have prompted caregivers to increase her water intake.

thirst

   b. The serum sodium of 156 mEq/L would indicate (hypo-, hyper-) natremia.

hyper-

   c. Her (low, normal, high) urine output was likely related to the high-protein feedings she was getting.

high

   d. Treatment would include (increasing, decreasing) her intake of water.

increasing

4. Betty was admitted to the hospital with a diagnosis of tachycardia. As you take a nursing history, you learn that Betty has been taking digoxin every morning for 12 years. She had rheumatic fever and then rheumatic heart disease, which resulted in congestive heart failure. Last week she had severe shortness of breath with very little activity, and her ankles were very edematous. Her physician gave her some "water pills" (diuretic), and she lost 25 pounds. Her serum potassium is 2.1 mEq/L.

low
    a. Betty's serum potassium is (low, normal, high).

3.5, 5
    b. The normal range for serum potassium is ___ to _ mEq/L.

    c. The probable cause for her hypokalemia is increased loss of potassium caused by increased urine output, which

diuretic
    was precipitated by the _____.

was
    d. Betty's tachycardia likely (was, was not) related to her hypokalemia.

    e. Treatment will include intravenous fluids that contain

potassium
    _____.

5. Bob, age 40, was admitted to the hospital with muscle weakness, abdominal cramps, and nausea. He has had no urine output for the past 24 hours. He has a history of chronic renal disease that began in childhood. His serum potassium is 7 mEq/L. His blood urea nitrogen (BUN) and creatinine are elevated.

hyperkalemia
    a. The electrolyte imbalance that Bob has is _____.

    b. The probable cause of the hyperkalemia is his
renal disease
    _____, which led to the lack of urine output.

    c. His nausea, abdominal cramps, and muscle weakness are
hyperkalemia
    likely caused by the _____.

    d. The major danger of a serum potassium level of 7 mEq/L
heart
    is its effect on Bob's ___.

T
    e. His ECG will show changes that include tall, peaked _ waves, widening of the QRS complex, and shortening of the Q-T interval.

    f. Since his situation is an emergency, one of the probable
hypertonic
    treatments will include intravenous (hypertonic, isotonic, hypotonic) glucose with insulin to help move potassium into the cells, followed by dialysis.

6. Mrs. Pizzingrilli was admitted to the hospital with regional enteritis accompanied by considerable diarrhea. She was given a bland diet plus a potassium supplement. She began to have periods of confusion and ataxia. Her deep tendon reflexes were hyperactive, and her Chvostek's sign was posi-

tive. She had a convulsion yesterday. Her serum potassium is normal. Her serum magnesium is 1 mEq/L.

a. Mrs. Pizzingrilli has an electrolyte imbalance called
_____.   hypomagnesemia

b. The probable cause for her low serum magnesium is impaired _____ because of the regional   intestinal absorption
enteritis.

c. The signs and symptoms can be explained by a lack of adequate _____.   magnesium

d. She is given magnesium sulfate intravenously. You should check her reflexes, respiratory rate, skin condition, and _____ every 5 to 10 minutes.   blood pressure

7. Mrs. Kryger, 52, has advanced chronic renal failure. She had gastric distress that was treated with a magnesium-containing antacid (Maalox). She has ECG changes, bradycardia, and decreased deep tendon reflexes. She has been lethargic and is now drowsy. Her serum magnesium is 7.5 mEq/L.

a. Mrs. Kryger's electrolyte imbalance is _____.   hypermagnesemia

b. You should expect that her use of the magnesium-containing antacid will be _____.   discontinued

c. The signs and symptoms can be explained by the
_____.   hypermagnesemia

d. A temporary measure that could be used to treat her would be intravenous _____, which has an   calcium gluconate
antagonistic effect on magnesium.

8. Mrs. Antonelli, 70, was admitted to the hospital because she has had a parasite for about 2 months. She has spent the past 10 years in the tropics, in the Amazon valley of Brazil. She has been having numerous large, foul-smelling stools daily. She complains of tingling and numbness in her fingers, abdominal cramps, and some memory loss. Physical assessment shows hyperactive reflexes and bilateral carpal spasms. Her serum calcium is 3.5 mEq/L.

a. Mrs. Antonelli's electrolyte imbalance is (hyper-, hypo-)   hypocalcemia.

b. The normal range for serum calcium is ___ to ___   8.5, 10.5
mEq/L.

c. Calcium is normally _____ through the GI tract.   absorbed

d. The signs and symptoms Mrs. Antonelli has can be explained by a lack of calcium, which leads to (increased, decreased) neuromuscular excitability.   increased

e. Important nursing interventions would include careful assessment, reporting of changes, and protection from
_____.   injury

9. Mr. Bucco, 54, began experiencing anorexia, then nausea and occasional vomiting. He became drowsy, lethargic, and unable to walk any distance. His daughter was especially concerned about his slurred speech and some brief periods of confusion. His serum electrolytes were bicarbonate 26 mEq/L and calcium 7.5 mEq/L. His parathyroid tests were normal. His urinalysis was normal except for the presence of numerous RBCs. An x-ray film revealed vascular changes in his right kidney. With further tests, a diagnosis of renal stenosis of the right kidney was made.

a. On the basis of his serum electrolytes, Mr. Bucco has

hypercalcemia

_____.

b. We know that the most common causes of hypercalcemia include excessive intake of calcium, vitamin D overdose,

release of calcium

and _____ from bone.

c. With the diagnosis of renal disease, Mr. Bucco's hypercalcemia could be explained by an interference with

renal resorption

_____.

10. Pat Ruane has had some diarrhea for the past 2 weeks, along with nausea and vomiting. Her weight has decreased significantly because she has been unable to eat or retain food. Pat has been very weak and unable to walk any distance. She has tremors in her hands and legs. On admission to the hospital, the significant laboratory results included a low RBC count, low hemoglobin, serum phosphorus of 1.2 mEq/L, and serum calcium of 5.5 mEq/L.

low

a. Ms. Ruane's phosphorus is (low, normal, high).

b. Her serum phosphorus of 1.2 mEq/L is called

hypophosphatemia

_____.

c. Her inability to eat and retain food for the past 2 weeks

contributed

(contributed, did not contribute) to her low phosphorus.

d. Ms. Ruane's signs and symptoms are consistent with

hypo-

(hyper-, hypo-) phosphatemia.

injury

e. Ms. Ruane could be at high risk for _____ related to muscular changes secondary to hypophosphatemia.

ASSESSMENT SUMMARY: FLUID, ACID-BASE, AND ELECTROLYTE IMBALANCE

TEMPERATURE

Increased: sodium excess, dehydration
Decreased: sodium deficit, fluid volume deficit

PULSE

Bounding: fluid excess
Easily obliterated: fluid deficit
Rapid, weak, thready: sodium deficit, fluid deficit
Weak, irregular, rapid: potassium deficit
Rapid: sodium excess
Dysrhythmias: potassium deficit and excess, magnesium deficit, respiratory acidosis and alkalosis, metabolic acidosis and alkalosis

NECK VEIN FILLING

Flat when supine: fluid deficit
Full when upright: fluid excess

CAPILLARY REFILL TIME

Increased: fluid deficit

RESPIRATION

Deep, rapid: metabolic acidosis, respiratory acidosis
Shallow, slow, irregular: metabolic alkalosis
Moist crackles: fluid excess
Shallow breathing: potassium deficit
Stridor: calcium deficit
Depressed: magnesium deficit

BLOOD PRESSURE

Hypotension: sodium deficit, potassium deficit, fluid deficit, magnesium deficit

Hypertension: fluid excess, magnesium deficit
Normal when lying flat and hypotension when head is elevated: fluid deficit

SKIN AND MUCOUS MEMBRANES

Poor skin turgor: fluid deficit
Flushed, dry skin: sodium excess, respiratory and metabolic acidosis
Cold, clammy skin: sodium deficit
Fingerprinting on sternum: sodium deficit
Rough, dry, red tongue: sodium excess
Dry mucous membranes with longitudinal wrinkles on tongue: fluid deficit
Tearing and salivation absent: fluid deficit

TENSENESS OF FONTANEL (INFANTS)

Bulging: fluid excess
Sunken: fluid deficit

WEIGHT

Gain: fluid excess
Loss: fluid deficit
2% of body weight = mild
5%-10% of body weight = moderate
10%-15% of body weight = severe

SPEECH

Difficulty forming words without first moistening tongue and lips: sodium excess, fluid deficit
Hoarseness: fluid deficit
Difficulty speaking because of muscular weakness: potassium deficit

BEHAVIOR

Lethargic: fluid deficit, magnesium excess
Impaired mental function: potassium deficit
Apprehension and giddiness: sodium deficit
Irritability, restlessness: potassium excess
Excitement (maniacal): sodium excess
Hallucinations: magnesium deficit
Confusion: fluid deficit, phosphorus deficit
Personality changes: sodium deficit, calcium excess

SKELETAL MUSCLES

Hypotonus: potassium deficit, calcium excess
Flabbiness: potassium deficit
Flaccid paralysis: potassium deficit or excess
Cramping of exercised muscles: calcium deficit, phosphorus excess
Muscle rigidity: calcium deficit
Chvostek's sign: calcium deficit, magnesium deficit
Convulsions: magnesium deficit, phosphorus excess
Trousseau's sign: calcium deficit, phosphorus excess

SENSATION

Tingling of fingers and toes: calcium deficit, potassium deficit, phosphorus excess
Light-headed: respiratory alkalosis
Abdominal cramps: sodium deficit, calcium deficit, potassium deficit and excess
Numb feeling: severe potassium deficit, potassium excess
Deep bony flank pain: calcium excess, phosphorus deficit
Nausea: potassium excess, sodium deficit, calcium excess, phosphorus excess
Abnormal sensitivity to sound: magnesium deficit
Dizziness when turned suddenly: sodium deficit

BIBLIOGRAPHY

1. Beare PG, Myers JL: *Adult health nursing*, ed 3, St Louis, 1998, Mosby.
2. Carlson-Catalano J and others: Clinical valuation of ineffective breathing pattern. Ineffective airway clearance and impaired gas exchange, *Image J Sch* 30(3):243, 1998.
3. Christensen B, Kockrow E: *Foundations of nursing*, ed 3, St Louis, 1998, Mosby.
4. Clayton BD, Stock YN: *Basic pharmacology for nurses*, ed 12, St Louis, 2001, Mosby.
5. Horne MM and others: *Mosby's pocket guide series: fluid, electrolyte, and acid-base balance*, ed 3, St Louis, 1997, Mosby.
6. Ignatavicius DD and others: *Medical-surgical nursing across the health care continuum*, ed 3, St Louis, 1999, Mosby.
7. Intravenous Nurses Society: Intravenous nursing standards of practice, *J Intraven Nurs* 21(15):535, 1998.
8. McCance KL, Huether SE: *Pathophysiology: the biologic basis for disease in adults and children*, ed 3, St Louis, 1998, Mosby.
9. McHenry LM, Salerno E: *Mosby's pharmacology in nursing*, ed 21, St Louis, 2001, Mosby.
10. Potter PA, Perry AG: *Basic nursing*, ed 4, St Louis, 1999, Mosby.
11. Potter PA, Perry AG: *Fundamentals of nursing*, ed 5, St Louis, 2001, Mosby.
12. Thompson JM and others: *Mosby's clinical nursing*, ed 4, St Louis, 1997, Mosby.
13. Wong DL, et al: *Whaley & Wong's nursing care of infants and children*, ed 6, St Louis, 1999, Mosby.
14. Wong DL, Hess CS: *Wong and Whaley's clinical manual of pediatric nursing*, ed 5, St Louis, 2000, Mosby.

INDEX

A

Acetoacetic acid, metabolic acidosis and, 95-96

Acid, hydrogen ion concentration and, 81

Acid-base balance/imbalance, 80-112, 99t

  assessment summary of, 191-193

  clinical conditions of, 92-101

    metabolic acidosis, 95-97, 96f, 97f

    metabolic alkalosis, 97-98, 98f

    respiratory acidosis, 92-94, 93f

    respiratory alkalosis, 94-95, 95f

  combination of types of, 98-99, 99t

  defense mechanisms, 84-92

    buffer system, 85-87

    renal system, 89-90

    respiratory system, 87-89

  effects of acidosis and alkalosis on the body, 99-101

  hydrogen ion concentration, 81-84

  nursing care in, 101-110

    blood gas analysis, 101-103

    general nursing responsibilities, 107-110

    metabolic origin, 104-107

    respiratory origin, 103-104

Acid-base regulatory mechanisms, 91t

Acidity, hydrogen ion concentration and, 81

Acidosis, 100

  central nervous system and, 108

  effects of, on body, 99-101

  hydrogen ion concentration and, 82

  metabolic, 95-97, 96f, 97f, 99t, 105, 139

  respiratory, 92-94, 93f, 99t, 103, 139

  respiratory system and, 88

Active transport, 12, 26, 116

Addison's disease, hyperkalemia and, 138

Adenosine triphosphate (ATP), 12, 26

  active transport and, 21

  hyperkalemia and, 145

  phosphorus imbalance and, 178

ADH; *see* Antidiuretic hormone (ADH)

Adolescents, fluid requirements for, 55

Adrenal cortical steroid hormones, hypokalemia and, 132

Adrenal glands, fluid and electrolyte balance and, 35

Adults

  average daily fluid gains and losses in, 28, 28t

  fluid requirements for, 55

  normal serum sodium in, 123

  proportion of body weight represented by fluid in, 5f

Alcoholism, hypomagnesemia and, 149

Aldactone; *see* Spironolactone (Aldactone)

Aldosterone

  fluid balance and, 34-35

  hypernatremia and, 126

  sodium imbalance and, 115

  urine volume and, 33

Alkaline antacids, hypercalcemia and, 172

Alkalinity, hydrogen ion concentration and, 81

Alkalosis, 99-100

  central nervous system and, 108

  effects of, on body, 99-101

  hydrogen ion concentration and, 83

  hypocalcemia and, 165-166

  metabolic, 97-98, 98f, 99t, 104, 105, 135

  respiratory, 94-95, 95f, 99t, 103, 104

Aluminum hydroxide gel, hyperphosphatemia and, 184

Aminophylline, respiratory alkalosis and, 95

195